THE
HEALING FACTOR
"Vitamin C"
Against Disease

THE
HEALING FACTOR

"Vitamin C"
Against Disease

Irwin Stone

GROSSET & DUNLAP
A National General Company

Publishers   New York

Produced in cooperation with
Whitehall, Hadlyme & Smith, Inc.

Foreword copyright © 1972 by Linus Pauling
Foreword copyright © 1972 by Albert Szent-Gyorgyi
Library of Congress Catalog Card Number: 72-77105
ISBN: 0-448-02130-7

Published simultaneously in Canada

Printed in the United States of America

This book is dedicated to my wife, Barbara, whose patience and collaboration over the years made it possible.

CONTENTS

The numerals set off in parentheses in the text are intended to guide the reader to the appropriate medical citation listed at the end of the book.

FOREWORD

by Linus Pauling

This is an important book—important to laymen, and important to physicians and scientists interested in the health of people.

Irwin Stone deserves much credit for having marshalled the arguments that indicate that most human beings have been receiving amounts of ascorbic acid less than those required to put them in the best of health. It is his contention, and it is supported by much evidence, that most people in the world have a disease involving a deficient intake of ascorbic acid, a disease that he has named *hypoascorbemia*. This disease seems to be present because of an evolutionary accident that occurred many millions of years ago. Ancestors of human beings (and of their close present-day relatives, other primates) were living in an area where the natural foods available provided very large amounts of ascorbic acid (very large in comparison with the amounts usually ingested now and the amounts usually recommended now by physicians and other authorities on nutrition). A mutation occurred that removed from the mutant the ability to manufacture ascorbic acid within his own body. Circumstances were such that the mutant had an evolutionary advantage over the other members of the population, who were burdened with the machinery for manufacturing additional ascorbic acid. The result was that the part of the population burdened with this machinery gradually died out, leaving the mutants, who depended upon their food for an adequate supply of ascorbic acid.

As man has spread over the earth and increased in number, the supplies of ascorbic acid have decreased. It is possible that most people in the world receive only one or two percent of the amounts of ascorbic acid that would keep them in the best of health. The resulting hypoascorbemia may be responsible for many of the illnesses that plague mankind.

In this book Irwin Stone summarizes the evidence. The publication of Irwin Stone's papers and of this book may ultimately result in a great improvement in the health of human beings everywhere, and a great decrease in the amount of suffering caused by disease.

Linus Pauling

FOREWORD

by Albert Szent-Gyorgyi, M.D., Ph.D.

My own interest in ascorbic acid centered around its role in vegetable respiration and defense mechanisms. All the same, I always had the feeling that not enough use was made of it for supporting human health. The reasons were rather complex. The medical profession itself took a very narrow and wrong view. Lack of ascorbic acid caused scurvy, so if there was no scurvy there was no lack of ascorbic acid. Nothing could be clearer than this. The only trouble was that scurvy is not a first symptom of lack but a final collapse, a premortal syndrome, and there is a very wide gap between scurvy and full health. But nobody knows what full health is! This could be found out by wide statistical studies, but there is no organization which could and would arrange such studies. Our society spends billions or trillions on killing and destruction but lacks the relatively modest means demanded to keep its own health and prime interest cared for. Full health, in my opinion, is the condition in which we feel best and show the greatest resistance to disease. This leads us into statistics which demand organization.

But there was also another, more individual difficulty. If you do not have sufficient vitamins and get a cold, and as a sequence pneumonia, your diagnosis will not be "lack of ascorbic acid" but "pneumonia." So you are waylaid immediately.

I think that mankind owes serious thanks to Irwin Stone for having kept the problem alive and having called Linus Pauling's attention to it.

On my last visit to Sweden, I was told that the final evidence has been found that ascorbic acid is quite harmless. An insane person had the fixed idea that he needed ascorbic acid so he swallowed incredible amounts of it for a considerable period without ill effects. So, apart from very specific conditions, ascorbic acid cannot hurt you. It does not hurt your pocket either, since it is very cheap. It is used for spraying trees.

I also fully agree with Dr. Pauling's contention that individual needs for vitamin C vary within wide limits. Some may need high doses, others may be able to get along with less, but the trouble is that you do not know to which group you belong. The symptoms of lack may be very different. I remember my correspondence with a teacher in my earlier days who told me that he had an antisocial boy whom he was unable to deal with. He gave him ascorbic acid and the boy became one of his most easygoing, obedient pupils. Nor does wealth and rich food necessarily protect against lack of vitamins. I remember my contact with one of the wealthiest royal families of Europe where the young prince had constant temperature and had poor health. On administering vitamin C, the condition readily cleared up.

It gives me great satisfaction to see this book appear and I hope very much that its message will be understood.

ACKNOWLEDGMENTS

This book took many years to write and involved many people. Because of a nonexistent budget and the fact that much of the data was in foreign languages, good friends had to be relied upon to supply translations. Among these friends were Lotte and George Bernard, Helene Gottlieb, Dorothy Kramer, Irving Minton, Jutta Nigrin, Sal Scaturo, Tanya Ronger, and Natasha and Otmar Silberstein.

Invaluable help and advice on library work were supplied by Eliphal Streeter and Vera Mitchell Throckmorton. The medical library of the Staten Island Public Health Hospital and the reprint facilities of the National Library of Medicine and the Medical Research Library of Brooklyn were especially helpful.

In any radically new scientific concept, encouragement and inspiration to carry on are difficult to come by. The author was fortunate in having men of scientific or medical stature such as Linus Pauling, Albert Szent-Gyorgyi, Frederick R. Klenner, Abram Hoffer, William J. McCormick, Thomas A. Garrett, Walter A. Schnyder, Louis A. Wolfe, Alexander F. Knoll, Marvin D. Steinberg, Benjamin Kramer, and A. Herbert Mintz as pillars of strength. Miriam T. Malakoff and Martin Norris supplied editorial advice and encouragement. My wife, Barbara, in the latter years, handled the bulk of the library research. To all these people and to many others who have contributed, go my deep gratitude and thanks. I trust that their efforts effectively contribute to better health for man.

Discovery consists in seeing
what everybody else has seen and
thinking what nobody has thought.
ALBERT SZENT-GYORGYI

INTRODUCTION

The purpose of this book is to correct an error in orientation which occurred in 1912, when ascorbic acid, twenty years before its actual discovery and synthesis, was designated as the trace nutrient, vitamin C. Thus, in the discussions in this book the terms "vitamin C" and "ascorbic acid" are identical, although the author prefers to use "ascorbic acid."

Scurvy, in 1912, was considered solely as a dietary disturbance. This hypothesis has been accepted practically unchallenged and has dominated scientific and medical thinking for the past sixty years. The purpose of this vitamin C hypothesis was to produce a rationale for the conquest of frank clinical scurvy. That it did and with much success, using minute doses of vitamin C. Frank clinical scurvy is now a rare disease in the developed countries because the amounts of ascorbic acid in certain foodstuffs are sufficient for its prevention. However, in the elimination of frank clinical scurvy, a more insidious condition, subclinical scurvy, remained; since it was less dramatic, it was glossed over and overlooked. Correction of subclinical scurvy needs more ascorbic acid than occurs naturally in our diet, requiring other non-dietary intakes. Subclinical scurvy i: the basis for many of the ills of mankind.

Because of this uncritical acceptance of a misaligned nutritional hypothesis, the bulk of the clinical research on the use of ascorbic acid in the treatment of diseases other than scurvy has been more like exercises in home economics than in the therapy of the sequelae of a fatal, genetic liver-enzyme disease. One of the objects of this book is to take the human physiology of ascorbic acid out of the dead-end of nutrition and put it where it belongs, in medical genetics. In medical genetics, wide vistas of preventive medicine and therapy are opened up by the full correction of this human error of carbohydrate metabolism.

For the past sixty years a vast amount of medical data has been collected relating to the use of ascorbic acid in diseases other than scurvy, but only very little practical therapeutic information has developed pertaining to its successful use in these diseases. The reader may well ask what is the difference between data and information? This can be illustrated by the following example: the number 382,436 is just plain data, but 38–24–36, that is information.

The most probable reason for the paucity of definitive therapeutic ascorbic acid information in the therapy of diseases other than scurvy is related to the fact that the vitamin C-oriented investigators were trying to relieve a trace-vitamin dietary disturbance and never used doses large enough to be pharmacologically and therapeutically effective. The new genetic concepts currently correct this old, but now obvious, mistake by supplying a logical rationale for these larger, pharmacologically effective treatments.

If the research suggestions contained in this book are properly and conscientiously followed through, it is the hope of the author that future medical historians may consider this as a major breakthrough in medicine of the latter quarter of the twentieth century.

While many scientific and medical papers have appeared, the publication of Dr. Linus Pauling's book, *Vitamin C and the Common Cold,* in late 1970, was the first scientific book ever published in the new medical fields of megascorbic prophylaxis and megascorbic therapy, which are branches of orthomolecular medicine. Dr. Pauling's book paved the way for this volume.

Since the size of the daily intake of ascorbic acid is so important in the later discussions, the reader can refer to the following table of equivalents. The dosages are usually expressed in the metric system in milligrams or grams of ascorbic acid:

Common Measures	Metric System Equivalents Milligrams	Grams
	1,000	1.0
1 ounce	28,350	28.35
½ teaspoonful*	1,500 to 2,000	1.5 to 2.0
20 international units	1	0.001

*teaspoons vary in size

PART I
Our Deadly Inheritance

1

THE BEGINNINGS OF LIFE

The first part of this book is a scientific detective story. The *corpus delicti* is a chemical molecule, and to collect the evidence in this case we have to cover billions of years in time and have to search in such odd places as frog kidneys, goat livers, and "cabbages and kings." The search will be rewarding because it will contribute to the understanding of this tremendously important molecule. The evidence we unearth will show that the lack of this molecule in humans has contributed to more deaths, sickness, and just plain misery than any other single factor in man's long history. When the molecule is finally discovered and assigned its rightful place in the scheme of things, and its potentialities for good are fully realized, undreamed-of vistas of exuberant health, freedom from disease, and long life will be opened up.

To start on the first leg of our journey, we will have to get into our Time Machine, set the dials, and go back 2.5 to 3 billion years. It will be necessary to seal ourselves completely in the Time Machine and carry a plentiful supply of oxygen because the atmosphere in those days was very different from what it is now. It will be hot and steamy, with little or no oxygen, and besides much water vapor, will contain notable quantities of gases such as carbon dioxide, methane, and ammonia. The hot seas will contain the products of the chemical experiments that Nature had been conducting for millions of years. If we are fortunate, we will arrive on the scene just as Nature was preparing to launch one of its most complicated and organized experiments—the production of living matter. If we were to sample the hot sea and examine it with our most powerful electron microscope, we would find in this thin consommé the culmination of these timeless chemical experiments in the form of a macromolecule having the property of being able to make exact duplicates of itself. The term "macromolecule" merely means a huge molecule which is formed out of a conglomeration of smaller unit molecules. The process of forming these huge molecules from the smaller units is called "polymerization," and is similar to building a brick wall (the macromolecule) from bricks (the smaller unit molecules). The "cement" holding the unit molecules together consists of various chemical and physical attractive forces of varying degrees of tenacity.

This self-reproducing macromolecule in this primordial soup might resemble some of our present-day viruses, but it had many important biochemical and biophysical problems to solve before it would begin to resemble some of the more primitive forms of life, such as bacteria, as we know them today. Nature had plenty of time to experiment and eventually came up with successful solutions to problems like heredity, enzyme formation, energy conservation, a protective covering for these naked macromolecules, and then cellular and multicellular organisms. The problem of heredity was solved so successfully by these early self-duplicating macromolecules that our present basis of heredity, the macromolecule DNA, is probably little changed from its original primordial form.

Enzyme formation was a problem that required an early solution if life was to continue evolving, since enzymes are the very foundation of the life process. An enzyme is a substance produced by a living organism which speeds up a specific chemical reaction. A chemical transformation that would require years to complete can be performed in moments by the mere presence of an enzyme. Enzymes are utilized by all living organisms to digest food, transform energy, synthesize tissues, and conduct nearly every biochemical reaction in the life process. The body contains thousands of enzymes.

Energy conservation and utilization was neatly solved in some of these early life forms by the development of photosynthesis: an enzymatic process which uses the energy of sunlight to transform carbon dioxide and water into carbohydrates. Carbohydrates are used for food and structural purposes, and these primitive forms evolved into the vast species of the plant kingdom.

At some time early in the development of life, certain primitive organisms developed the enzymes needed to manufacture a unique substance that offered many solutions to the multiple biological problems of survival. This compound, ascorbic acid, is a relatively simple one compared to the many other huge, complicated molecules produced by living organisms. Because of its unique properties, however, it is somewhat unstable and transient, a fact that will complicate our later search for this substance.

We now know that ascorbic acid is a carbohydrate derivative containing six carbon atoms, six oxygen atoms, and eight hydrogen atoms and is closely related to the sugar, glucose (see Figure 1). Glucose is of almost universal occurrence in living organisms, where it is used as a prime source of energy. Ascorbic acid is produced enzymatically from this sugar in both plants and animals.

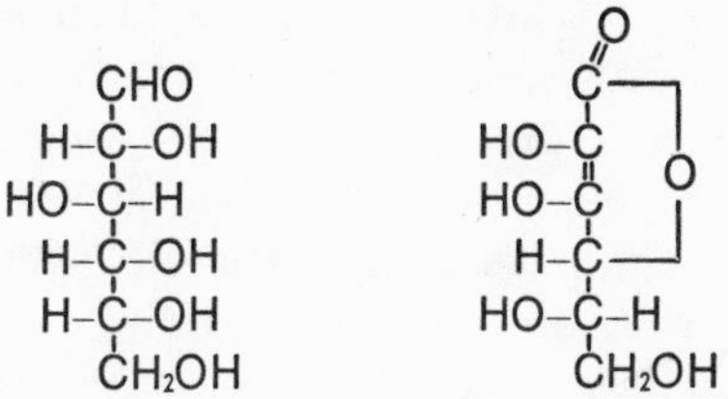

Figure 1

Glucose

Ascorbic
Acid

We can surmise that the production of ascorbic acid was an early accomplishment of the life process because of its wide distribution in nearly all present-day living organisms. It is produced in comparatively large amounts in the simplest plants and the most complex; it is synthesized in the most primitive animal species as well as in the most highly organized. Except possibly for a few microorganisms, those species of animals that cannot make their own ascorbic acid are the exceptions and require it in their food if they are to survive. Without it, life cannot exist. Because of its nearly universal presence in both plants and animals we can also assume that its production was well organized before the time when evolving life forms diverged along separate plant and animal lines.

This early development of the ascorbic acid synthesizing mechanisms probably arose from the need of these primitive living organisms to capture electrons from an environment with very low levels of oxygen. This process of scavenging for rare oxygen was a great advance for the survival and development of the organisms so equipped. It also may have triggered the development of the photosynthetic process and sparked the tremendous development of plant life. This great increase in plant life, with its use of the energy of sunlight to produce oxygen and remove carbon dioxide from the atmosphere, completely changed the chemical composition of the atmosphere, over a period of possibly a billion years, from oxygen-free air which would not support living animals as we know them to a life-giving oxygen supply approaching the composition of our present atmosphere.

The increase in the oxygen content of the atmosphere had other, important consequences. In the upper reaches of the atmosphere, oxygen is changed by radiation into ozone, which is a more active form of oxygen. This layer of high-altitude ozone acts as a filter to remove the deadly ultraviolet rays from sunlight and makes life on land possible. This series of events, which occurred more than 600 million years ago, preceded the tremendous forward surge of life and the development of more complicated, multicellular organisms in post-Cambrian times, as is seen in the fossil record.

The only living organisms that survive to this day in a form that has not progressed or evolved much from the forms which existed in the earliest infra-Cambrian times are primitive single-cell organisms, such as bacteria, which do not make (and may not need) ascorbic acid in their living environment. All plants or animals which have evolved into complex multicellular forms make or need ascorbic acid. Was ascorbic acid the stimulus for the evolution of multicellular organisms? If not the stimulus, it certainly increased the biochemical adaptability necessary for survival in changing and unfavorable environments.

Further evidence for the great antiquity of the ascorbic acid-synthesizing systems may be obtained from the science of embryology. During its rapid fetal development, the embryo passes through the various evolutionary stages that its species went through in time. This led nineteenth-century embryologists to coin the phrase, "ontogeny recapitulates phylogeny," which is another way of saying the same thing. In fetal development, ascorbic acid can be detected very early, when the embryo is nothing more than a shapeless mass of cells. For instance, in the development of the chick embryo (which is convenient to work with), the chicken egg is devoid of ascorbic acid, but it can be detected in the early blastoderm stage of the growing embryo. At this stage the embryo is just a mass of cells in which no definite organs have as yet appeared, and it resembles the most primitive multicellular organisms—both fossil and present living forms. In plants, also, the seeds have no ascorbic acid, but as soon as the plant embryo starts to develop, ascorbic acid is immediately formed. Thus all the available evidence points to the great antiquity of the ascorbic acid-synthesizing systems in life on this planet.

2

FROM FISHES TO MAMMALS

If we reset the dials in our Time Machine and travel to a point about 450 million years ago, we may be able to witness the start of another notable experiment by Nature. In the seas are the beginnings of the vertebrates, a long line of animals that will eventually evolve into the mammals and man. These are the animals with a more or less rigid backbone, containing the start of a well-organized and complex nervous and muscular system, and capable of reacting much more efficiently to their environment than the swarms of simpler, spineless invertebrates, which had apparently reached the end of their evolutionary rope. Nature was ready to embark on another revolutionary, and more complicated, experiment.

Because of the increased complexity of their nervous system and a fast-acting muscular system, these primitive vertebrate fishes were able to gather food better and avoid enemies and other perils, all of which had increased survival value. Before they could do this, however, they had to develop complex, specialized organ systems in which various biochemical processes were carried out. And their requirements for ascorbic acid were undoubtedly much higher because of their much increased activity. The simpler structures of the invertebrates no longer sufficed and required much modification to suit the needs of these more active and alert upstarts, the vertebrates.

The vertebrate fishes were such a successful evolutionary experiment that for the next 100 million years or so they dominated the waters. Nature was now ready to carry out another experiment—that of taking the animals out of the crowded seas and putting them on dry land. It had experience in this sort of operation since the plants had long ago left the seas and were well established on land. The land was no longer a place of barren fields, but was covered with dense vegetation. Two lines of modification were tried: in one, the fish was structurally modified so that it could clumsily exist out of the water; in the other, a more complete renovation job was done. Modifications of the fins and the swim bladder ended in the evolutionary blind alley of the lung fishes, but the more ambitious program—involving a complete change in the biochemistry and life cycle—produced a more successful line—the amphibians. These creatures are born in the water and spend their early life there and then they metamorphose into land-living forms. Frogs and salamanders are present-day denizens of this group. The next step in evolution was to produce wholly land-living animals—the reptiles. These were scaly animals that slithered, crawled, walked, or ran; and some grew to prodigious size. Some preferred swimming and reverted to the water and others took to the air. It was these airborne species that eventually evolved into the warm-blooded birds. The birds are of particular interest to us because they solved an ascorbic acid problem in the same fashion as the primitive mammals, which were appearing on the scene at about this time.

We have gone into this cursory sketch of this period of evolutionary history to trace the possible history of ascorbic acid in these ancient animals. If we assume that the present-day representatives of the amphibians, the reptiles, the birds, and the mammals have the same biochemical systems as their remote ancestors, then we can do some more detective work on our elusive molecule. These complex vertebrates all have well-defined organ systems that are assigned certain definite functions. Usually an organ has a main biological function and also many other accessory, but no less important, biochemical responsibilities. The kidney, whose main function is that of selective filtration and excretion, is also the repository of enzyme systems for the production of vitally important chemicals needed by the body. The liver, which is the largest organ of the body, functions mainly to neutralize poisons, produce bile, and act as a storage depot for carbohydrate reserves; but it also has many other duties to perform.

In examining present-day creatures we find that in the fishes, amphibians, and reptiles, the place where ascorbic acid is produced in the body is localized in the kidney. When we investigate the higher vertebrates, the mammals, we find that the liver is the production site and the kidneys are inactive. Apparently, during the course of evolution the production of enzymes for the synthesis of ascorbic acid was shifted from the small, biochemically crowded kidneys to the more ample space of the liver. This shift was the evolutionary response to the needs of the more highly developed species for greater supplies of this vital substance.

The birds are of particular interest because they illustrate this transition. In the older orders of the birds, such as the chickens, pigeons, and owls, the enzymes for synthesizing ascorbic acid are in the kidneys. In the more recently evolved species, such as the mynas and the song birds, both the kidneys and the liver are sites of synthesis; and in other species only the liver is active and the kidneys are no longer involved in the manufacture of ascorbic acid. Thus we have a panoramic picture of this evolutionary change in the birds, where the process has been "frozen" in their physiology for millions of years.

This evolutionary shift from the kidneys to the liver took place at a time when temperature regulatory mechanisms were evolving and warm-blooded animals were developing from the previous, cold-blooded vertebrates. In the cold-blooded amphibians and reptiles, the amounts of ascorbic acid that were produced in their small kidneys sufficed for their needs. However, as soon as temperature regulatory means were evolved—producing the highly active, warm-blooded mammals—the biochemically crowded kidneys could no longer supply ascorbic acid in ample quantities. Both the birds and the mammals, the two concurrently evolving lines of vertebrates, independently arrived at the same solution to their physiological problem: the shift to the liver.

3

OUR ANCESTRAL PRIMATE

If we come forward to a time some 55 to 65 million years ago we will find that the warm-blooded vertebrates are the dominant animals, and they are getting ready to evolve into forms that are familiar to us. Life has come a long way since it discovered how to make ascorbic acid. In the warmer areas the vegetation is dense and the ancestors of our present-day primates— the monkeys, apes, and man—shared the forests and treetops with the innumerable birds.

At about this time something very serious happened to a common ancestor of ours, the animal who would be a progenitor of some of the present primates. This animal suffered a mutation that eliminated an important enzyme from its biochemical makeup. The lack of this enzyme could have proved deadly to the species and we would not be here to read about it except for a fortuitous combination of circumstances.

Perhaps we should digress here and review some facts of mammalian biochemistry as related to this potentially lethal genetic

15

accident. It will not be difficult, and it will help in understanding the thesis of this book.

All familiar animals are built from billions of cells. Masses of cells form the different tissues, the tissues form organs, and the whole animal is a collection of organs. The cell is the ultimate unit of life. Each cell has a cell membrane, which separates it from neighboring cells and encloses a jellylike mass of living stuff. Floating in this living matter is the nucleus, which is something like another, smaller cell within the cell. This nucleus contains the reproducing macromolecule called desoxyribonucleic acid (DNA). DNA is the biochemical basis of heredity and determines whether the growing cells will develop into an oak tree, a fish, a man or whatever. This molecule is a long, thin, double-stranded spiral containing linear sequences of four different basic unit molecules. The sequence of the four unit molecules as they are arranged on this spiral is the code that forms the hereditary blueprint of the organism. When a cell divides, this double-stranded molecule separates into two single strands and each daughter cell receives one. In the daughter cell, the single strand reproduces an exact copy of itself to again form the double strand and in this way each cell contains a copy of the hereditary pattern of the organism.

These long threadlike molecules are coiled and form bodies in the nucleus that were called chromosomes by early microscopists because they avidly absorbed dyes and stains and thus became readily visible in preparations viewed microscopically. These microscopists suspected that these bodies were in some way connected with the process of inheritance but did not know the exact mechanisms.

Certain limited sections of these long, spiral molecules, which direct or control a single property such as the synthesis of a single enzyme, are called genes. A chromosome may be made up of thousands of genes. The exact order of the four different unit molecules in a gene determines, say, the protein structure of an enzyme. If only one of these unit molecules is out of place or transposed among the thousands in a gene sequence, the protein structure of the enzyme will be modified and its enzymatic activity may be changed or destroyed. Such a change in the sequence of a DNA molecule is called a mutation.

These mutations can be produced experimentally by means of various chemicals and by radiations such as X rays, ultraviolet rays, or gamma rays. Cosmic rays, in nature, are no doubt a factor in inducing mutations. It is on these mutations that Nature has depended to produce changes in evolving organisms. If the mutation is favorable and gives the plant or animal an advantage in survival, it is transmitted to its descendants. If it is unfavorable and produces death before reproduction takes place, the mutation dies out with the mutated individual and is regarded as a lethal mutation. Some unfavorable mutations which are serious enough to be lethal, but which the mutated animal survives, are called conditional lethal mutations. This type of mutation struck a primitive monkey that was the ancestor of man and some of our present-day primates.

In nearly all the mammals, ascorbic acid is manufactured in the liver from the blood sugar, glucose. The conversion proceeds stepwise, each step being controlled by a different enzyme. The mutation that occurred in our ancestral monkey destroyed his ability to manufacture the last enzyme in this series—L-gulonolactone oxidase. This prevented his liver from converting L-gulonolactone into ascorbic acid, which was needed to carry out the various biochemical processes of life. The lack of this enzyme made this animal susceptible to the deadly disease, scurvy. To this day, millions of years later, all the descendants of this mutated animal, including man, have the intermediate enzymes but lack the last one. And that is why man cannot make ascorbic acid in his liver.

This was a serious mutation because organisms without ascorbic acid do not last very long. However, by a fortuitous combination of circumstances, the animal survived. First of all, the mutated animal was living in a tropical or semitropical environment where fresh vegetation, insects, and small animals were available the year round as a food supply. All these are good dietary sources of ascorbic acid. Secondly, the amount of ascorbic acid needed for mere survival is low and could be met from these available sources of food. This is not to say that this animal was getting as much ascorbic acid from its food as it would have produced in its own body if it had not mutated. While the amount may not have been optimal, it was sufficient to ward off death from scurvy. Under these ideal conditions the mutation was not serious enough to have too adverse an effect on survival. It was only later when this animal's descendants moved from these ideal surroundings, this

Garden of Eden, and became "civilized" that they—we—ran into trouble.

This defective gene has been transmitted for millions of years right up to the present-day primates. This makes man and a few other primates unique among the present-day mammals. Nearly all other mammals manufacture ascorbic acid in their livers in amounts sufficient to satisfy their physiological requirements. This had great survival value for these mammals, who, when subjected to stress, were able to produce much larger amounts of ascorbic acid to counteract adverse biochemical effects. And there was plenty of stress for an animal living in the wild, competing for scarce food, and trying to avoid becoming a choice morsel for some other predator.

To the best of our knowledge, only two other non-primate mammals have suffered a similar mutation and have survived. How many others may have similarly mutated and died off, we shall never know. The guinea pig survived in the warm lush forests of New Guinea where vegetation rich in fresh ascorbic acid was readily available. The other mammal is a fruit-eating bat *(Pteropus medius)* from India. The only other vertebrates that are known to harbor this defective gene are certain passeriforme birds.

Because of this missing or defective gene, man, some of the other primates, the guinea pig, and a bat will develop and die of scurvy if deprived of an outside source of ascorbic acid. A guinea pig, for example, will die a horrible death within two weeks if totally deprived of ascorbic acid in its diet.

4

THE EVOLUTION OF MAN

In the last chapter it was estimated that the conditional lethal mutation which destroyed our ancestral monkey's ability to produce his own ascorbic acid occurred some 55 to 65 million years ago. Actually, we do not know which primate ancestor was afflicted with this mutation, nor can we exactly pinpoint this occurrence in the time scale. Up to the time of this writing, little work has been done to try to obtain this important data. However, for the purposes of our discussion, it is not essential to know exactly which of man's ancestors was burdened with this genetic defect nor when it happened. It is sufficient to know that it happened before man came on the scene. Presently available evidence indicates that the members of the primate suborder Anthropoidea, the old world monkeys, the new world monkeys, the apes and man, still carry this defective gene.

While this defect did not wipe out the mutated species, it must have put these animals at a serious disadvantage. Normally, a mammal equipped to synthesize its own ascorbic acid will produce it in variable amounts depending upon the stresses the animal is undergoing. These animals have a feedback mechanism that produces more when the animal needs more. The stresses of living under wild and unfavorable conditions were great. The animals had to continually keep out of the way of predators while they searched for food; they had to procreate and take care of their young; they had to resist such environmental stresses as heat, cold, rain, and snow, and the biological stresses of parasites and diseases of bacterial, fungal, and viral origin. Animals that were able to cope with these stresses by producing optimal amounts of ascorbic acid within their bodies were more resistant to environmental extremes of heat and cold, better able to fight off infections and disease, better able to recover from physical trauma, and better prepared to do it repeatedly. The presence of the ascorbic acid-synthesizing enzymes conferred enormous powers of survival.

It is likely that our mutated ancestors never got enough ascorbic acid from their food to completely combat all the biochemical stresses. It is equally certain that the amounts they ingested were enough to insure their survival until they were able to reproduce and raise their young. Their genetic defect must surely have been a serious handicap in their fight for survival, but they did survive.

If we follow the trunk of the evolving primate tree, we come to animals that we know from their fossil remains. *Propliopithecus, Proconsul, Oreopithecus,* and *Ramapithecus,* to name a few, may have been the ancestors of the present-day higher primates. These animals were more ape than man, but we are coming closer. About a million years ago we find *Australopithecus* of Southern Africa. These creatures were no longer living an arboreal existence, swinging through the branches of the forest; they had come down to earth and lived in the wide-open spaces of the grassy plains. While in appearance they still resembled chimpanzees, they held their heads erect, not thrust forward; and they were built to walk erect most of the time. Their hands had fingers too slender to walk upon and their jaws contained teeth more human-like.

In the last million years, evolution developed recognizably human forms. Heidelberg man, *Pithecanthropus, Sinanthropus,* Swanscombe man, and others bring us to a point about 100,000 years ago. From here on we find the remains of manlike creatures widely distributed: Neanderthal man in the Near East and Europe; Rhodesian man in South Africa; and later, 20,000 to 40,000 years ago, modern man in Europe, Asia, South Africa, and America. The Neanderthal man of 50,000 to 70,000 years ago was a great hunter and went after the biggest and fiercest animals, the woolly rhinoceroses and mammoths. Appetites and diets evolved from the vegetation, fruits, nuts, and insects of the arboreal monkeys, to the raw red meat of these primitive hunters. Fresh raw meat is a good source of ascorbic acid, and Neanderthal man needed plenty of it to survive the climate that had started to turn cold, and the glaciers that covered most of Europe about 50,000 years ago. From a study of a Neanderthal skeleton found in France about a half century ago, it was concluded that Neanderthal man did not stand erect but walked with knees bent in an uncertain, shuffling gait. However, it was later discovered that this skeleton was that of an older man with a severe case of arthritis—fossil evidence of a pattern which might indicate the lack of sufficient ascorbic acid to overcome the stresses of Ice-Age cold and infection.

The evolution of the nervous system and the explosive development of the brain and intelligence compensated in some measure for this biochemical defect by finding new sources of ascorbic acid. The normally herbivorous and insect-eating species became hunters after raw red meat and fish, and later went on to raise their own animals. It was this change in dietary practice that permitted the wide dispersion of the humanoids. They were no longer limited to tropical or semitropical areas where plants or insects rich in ascorbic acid were available the year round. To gauge the effect of this factor, just compare the wide dispersion of man on the face of this globe with his less adaptable primate relatives, the monkeys and apes. They are still swinging in the branches close to their supply of ascorbic acid.

This dispersal of primitive man into environs for which he was not biochemically adapted was not easy and was only accomplished at a high cost—increased mortality, shortened life span, and great physical suffering. Man's survival under these unfavorable conditions is a tribute to his guts and brainpower. Here was one of Nature's first experiences with an organism that could fight back against an unfavorable environment and win. But the victory, as we can see all around us, was a conditional one.

A study of the remains found in ancient burial grounds reveals some of the privations suffered by Stone Age man and his descendants. Living in the temperate zone, the cold was a constant threat to his existence. The exhumed bones give evidence of much disease, nutritional deficiencies, and general starvation. Infant and child mortality was enormous, and the life span of those who survived their teens was rarely beyond thirty or thirty-five years. Some abnormalities evidenced in the fossilized limbs of these ancient populations could have been caused by recurring episodes of inadequate intake of ascorbic acid. Future studies in paleopathology should bring additional interesting facts to light.

Another way of assessing the extent of the ascorbic acid nutriture of these ancient peoples is to find out what current primitive societies used as food, and what their methods of food preparation and preservation were before "civilization" reached them: the Australian aborigine, the native tribes of Africa, the Indians of the Americas, and the Eskimo, who has worked out a pattern for survival in a most unfavorable environment.

In reviewing the diets of these peoples, one is impressed by their variety. All products of the plant and animal kingdoms, without exception, were at one time or another consumed. Those who ate their food fresh and raw had more chance of obtaining ascorbic acid. Extended cooking or drying tends to destroy ascorbic acid. The availability of food appears to have been the main factor in an individual's nutrition and, aside from certain tribal taboos, there were no aesthetic qualms against eating any kind of food. A luscious spider's abdomen bitten off and eaten raw, a succulent lightly toasted locust consumed like a barbecued shrimp, the larva of the dung beetle soaked in coconut milk and roasted were good sources of ascorbic acid. Similarly, raw fish, seaweed, snails, and every variety of marine mollusk were tasty morsels for those peoples living near the shores.

The name "Eskimo" comes from the Cree Indian word "uskipoo," meaning "he eats raw meat." During the long winter, Eskimos depended upon the ascorbic acid content of raw fish or freshly caught raw seal meat and blood. Any Eskimo who cooked his fish and meat—thereby reducing its ascorbic acid content— would never have survived long enough to tell about his newfangled technique of food preparation. But not even the best of these diets ever supplied ascorbic acid in the amounts that would have been produced in man's own liver if he had the missing gene. The levels were, as always, greatly submarginal for optimal health and longevity, especially under high-stress conditions. The estimated life expectancy for an Eskimo man in northern Greenland is only twenty-five years.

Two great advances in the early history of man were the development of agriculture and the domestication of animals. In the temperate zones, agriculture tended to concentrate on cereal grains or other seed crops, which could easily be stored without deterioration and used during the long winters. These crops are notably lacking in ascorbic acid and, while they supplied calories, scurvy would soon develop in those who depended on them as a staple diet. Whatever fresh vegetables or fruits were grown were generally rendered useless as an antiscorbutic foodstuff for winter use by the primitive methods of drying and preservation.

A trick for imparting antiscorbutic qualities to seed crops was discovered by various agricultural peoples and then forgotten. It was rediscovered again in Germany in 1912, and it has persisted among some Asiatic people. This simple life-saving measure was to take portions of these seed crops (beans and the like), soak them in water, and then allow them to germinate and sprout. The sprouted seeds were consumed. Ascorbic acid is required by the growing plant and it is one of the first substances that is synthesized in the growing seed to nourish the plant embryo. Bean sprouts are even now a common item of the Chinese cuisine as they have been for thousands of years; they contain our elusive molecule, while unsprouted beans do not.

The early people whose culture was based upon animal husbandry may have fared better in the winter than the agricultural people. They had a built-in continuous ascorbic acid supply in their fresh milk, fresh meat, and blood. If they used these products fresh they were safe, but if they attempted long preservation, the antiscorbutic properties were lost and the foodstuffs became potential poisons.

All in all, it has been a terrible struggle throughout prehistory and history to obtain the little daily speck of ascorbic acid required for mere survival.

5

FROM PREHISTORY TO THE EIGHTEENTH CENTURY

Now we come to man in historical times and find that he has been plagued by the effects of this genetic defect from the earliest days of recorded history. Before discussing this great scourge of mankind, let us examine the disease caused by this genetic defect. Clinical scurvy is such a loathsome and fatal affliction that it is difficult to conceive that an amount of ascorbic acid that could be piled upon the head of a pin is enough to prevent its fatal effects.

In describing the disease we must distinguish between chronic scurvy and acute scurvy. Chronic or biochemical scurvy is a disease that practically everyone suffers from and its individual severity depends upon the amount of one's daily intake of ascorbic acid. It is a condition where the normal biochemical processes of the body are not functioning at optimal levels because of the lack of sufficient ascorbic acid. There are all shades of biochemical scurvy and it can vary from a mild "not feeling right" to conditions where one's resistance is greatly lowered and susceptibility to disease, stress, and trauma is increased. The chronic form usually exists without showing the clinical signs of the acute form and this makes it difficult to detect and diagnose without special biochemical testing procedures. The acute form is the "classical" scurvy recognized from ancient times and is due to prolonged deprivation of ascorbic acid, usually combined with severe stress.

The first symptom of acute scurvy in an adult is a change in complexion: the color becomes sallow or muddy. There is a loss of accustomed vigor, increased lassitude, quick tiring, breathlessness, a marked disinclination for exertion, and a desire for sleep. There may be fleeting pains in the joints and limbs, especially the legs. Very soon the gums become sore, bleed readily, and are congested and spongy. Reddish spots (small hemorrhages) appear on the skin, especially on the legs at the sites of hair follicles. Sometimes there are nosebleeds or the eyelids become swollen and purple or the urine contains blood. These signs progress steadily—the complexion becomes dingy and brownish, the weakness increases, with the slighest exertion causing palpitation and breathlessness. The gums become spongier and bleed, the teeth become loose and may fall out, the jawbone starts to rot, and the breath is extremely foul. Hemorrhages into any part of the body may ensue. Old healed wounds and scars on the body may break open and fresh wounds and sores show no tendency to heal. Pains in the limbs render the victim helpless. The gums swell so much that they overlap and hide the teeth and may protrude from the mouth. The bones become so brittle that a leg may be broken by merely moving in bed. The joints become so disorganized that a rattling noise can be heard from the bones grating against each other when the patient is moved. Death usually comes rapidly from sudden collapse at slight exertion or from a secondary infection, such as pneumonia. This sequence of events, from apparent health to death, may take only a few months.

Acute clinical scurvy was recognized early by ancient physicians and was probably known long before the dawn of recorded history. Each year in the colder climes, as winter closed in, the populations were forced onto a diet of cereal grains and dried or salted meat or fish, all low in ascorbic acid. Foods rich in ascorbic acid were scarce if not entirely lacking. The consequence of this inadequate diet was that near the end of winter and in early spring, whole populations were becoming increasingly scorbutic. Thus weakened, their resistance low, people were easy prey for the rampant bacterial and viral infections that decimated the population. This happened year after year for centuries and this is the origin of the so-called "spring tonics," which were attempts to alleviate this annually recurring scurvy (by measures which were generally ineffective). The number of lives lost in this annual debacle and the toll in human misery are inestimable. People became so accustomed to this recurring catastrophe that it was looked upon as the normal course of events and casually accepted as such. Only in times of civil strife, of wars and sieges, or on long voyages, where the toll in lives lost to this dread disease was so great, did it merit special notice.

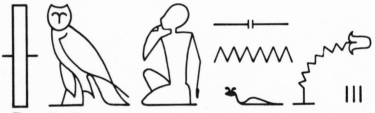

Figure 2   Egyptian hieroglyphs believed to indicate scurvy

The earliest written reference to a condition that is recognizable as scurvy is in the Ebers papyrus, a record of Egyptian medical lore written about 1500 B.C. Figure 2 shows various Egyptian hieroglyphs for scurvy. The figure of the little man pointing to his mouth and the lips oozing blood indicated the bleeding gums of the disease. It is likely that scurvy was clearly recognized at least 3,000 years ago. Hippocrates (ca. 400 B.C.), the father of medicine, described diseases that sound suspiciously like scurvy. Pliny the Elder (A.D. 23–79), in his *Natural History,* describes a disease of Roman soldiers in Germany whose symptoms bespeak of scurvy and which was cured by a plant *herba Britannica.* Sire Jean de Joinville, in his history of the invasion of Egypt by the Crusaders of Saint Louis in 1260, gives a detailed description of the scurvy that afflicted this army. He mentions the hemorrhagic spots, the fungous and putrid gums, and the legs being affected. It was scurvy that led to the ultimate defeat and capture of Saint Louis and his knights. It is certain that, throughout the Crusades, scurvy took a far greater toll of the Crusaders than all the weapons of the Saracens.

In the great cycle of epidemics that hit Europe in the fourteenth century—the Black Death of the Middle Ages—millions of people died. The Black Death was a fulminating, virulent epidemic of a bacterial disease, bubonic plague, concurrent with pulmonary infection superimposed on scurvy with its diffused superficial hemorrhages that caused the skin to turn black or bluish-black. The fact that the disease attacked a population that was first thoroughly weakened by scurvy accounts for the extremely high mortality: one-fourth of the population of Europe—or 25 million deaths. It is known that resistance to infection is lowered by a deficiency of ascorbic acid, so a disease which would normally be a mild affliction could whip through a scorbutic population with unprecedented fierceness and fatally strike down thousands.

With the invention of the printing press and the easier dissemination of the printed word, the sixteenth and following centuries saw the appearance of many tracts that described scurvy and its bizarre causes, and offered many different exotic treatments and "cures" for the disease. Much earlier, folklore had associated scurvy with a lack of fresh foodstuffs, and the antiscorbutic qualities of many plants had been known. But these qualities were forgotten and had to be rediscovered again and again at great cost in lives and suffering.

Improved ship construction and the ensuing long voyages provided ideal conditions for the rapid development of acute scurvy under circumstances where the developing symptoms could be readily observed and recorded. Sailors quickly succumbed to scurvy due to inadequate diet; physical exertions; exposure to extremes of heat, cold, and dampness; and the generally unsanitary shipboard conditions. In a few short months, out of what started off as a seemingly healthy crew, only a few remained fit for duty and were able to stand watch. The logs of these voyages make incredible reading today. Before scurvy was finally controlled, this scourge destroyed more sailors than all other causes, including the extremely high tolls of naval warfare.

In 1497, Vasco da Gama, while attempting to find a passage to the Indies by way of the Cape of Good Hope, lost 100 of his 160-man crew to scurvy. Magellan, in 1519, set sail with a fleet of five ships on one of history's great voyages, the circumnavigation of the earth. Three years later, only one ship, with only eighteen members of the original crew, returned to Spain. On occasion, a Spanish galleon would be found drifting, a derelict, its entire crew dead of scurvy. Many books were written on scurvy during the sixteenth to eighteenth centuries; some authors hit upon means to actually combat the disease, while others, clouded by the medical lore of the times, were way off base.

We still find logs of eighteenth-century voyages that recount the devastating effects of scurvy, and others where the master of the ship was able to prevent the disease. In 1740, Commodore Anson left England with six vessels and 1500 seamen; he returned four years later with one ship and 335 men. Between 1772 and 1775, on his round-the-world trip, however, Captain James Cook lost only one man out of his crew of 118, and that one not from scurvy. Cook took every opportunity when touching land to obtain supplies of fresh vegetables and fruit. He usually had a good store of sauerkraut aboard and he knew the beneficial qualities of celery and scurvy grass. After the voyage was completed, Cook was presented with the Copley Medal of the Royal Society. This award was given for his success in making such a lengthy voyage without a single death from scurvy—not for his great navigational and geographic discoveries. His scientific contemporaries understood the great significance of Cook's accomplishment. Between the time of Anson's failure and Cook's great success another important event took place; the first modern type of medical experiment was carried out by James Lind. We will discuss this later.

This is only a very brief record of the easily avoidable havoc caused by scurvy on the high seas, but those on land fared little better. In addition to the fearful, annually recurring scorbutic devastation of the population in the late winter and early spring, there were special circumstances which brought on deadly epidemics of acute scurvy. Wars and long sieges brought these epidemics to a head. In a brief sampling of the wars of the sixteenth to eighteenth century, scurvy appeared at the siege of Breda in Holland in 1625 and at Thorn in Prussia in 1703, where it accounted for 5,000 deaths among the garrison and noncombatants. It took its toll of the Russian armies in 1720 in the war between the Austrians and the Turks, of the English troops that captured Quebec in 1759, and of the French soldiers in the Alps in the spring of 1795.

Witness also Jacques Cartier's expedition to Newfoundland in 1535. These were men from a civilized culture with a long background of medical lore. One hundred of Cartier's 110 men were dying of scurvy until the Indian natives showed him how to make a decoction from the tips of the spruce fir which cured his men. This trick, incidentally, was also used by the defenders of Stalingrad in Word War II to stave off scurvy.

By the middle of the eighteenth century, the stage had been prepared for advances in the prevention and treatment of scurvy. Admiral Sir Richard Hawkins, in 1593, protected the crew of the *Dainty* with oranges and lemons; among others, Commodore Lancaster, in voyages for the East India Company, had shown by 1600 that scurvy was an easily preventable disease. It remained, however, for James Lind to prove this. James Lind, surgeon's mate on H.M.S. *Salisbury,* was inspired by the hardships of the Anson fiasco and the many cases of scurvy he had treated on his own ships. Lind was a keen observer and eventually became known as "the father of nautical medicine." He conducted the first properly controlled clinical therapeutic trial on record.

The crucial experiment Lind performed in 1747 at sea on the *Salisbury* was to take twelve seamen suffering from the same degree of scurvy and divide them into six groups of two each. In addition to their regular diet, he gave each group a different, commonly used treatment for scurvy and observed its action. One group received a quart of cider daily, the second group received twenty-five drops of dilute sulfuric acid three times a day, the third group was given two spoonfuls of vinegar three times a day, the fourth team drank half a pint of seawater three times a day, the fifth received a concoction of garlic, mustard seed, horseradish, gum myrrh, and balsam of Peru. The last group received two oranges and one lemon daily for six days. These last two men improved with such astonishing rapidity that they were used as nurses to care for the others. There was slight improvement in the cider group but no benefit was observed in the others. Here was clear-cut, easily understandable evidence of the value of citrus fruit in the cure of scurvy. Although Lind did not realize it, he had found a good natural source of our elusive molecule.

Lind left the Royal Navy in 1748, obtained an M.D. degree from Edinburgh University, and went into private practice. He was later physician at the Royal Naval Hospital at Haslar and physician to the Royal Household of George III at Windsor. He continued his work on scurvy and, in 1753, published one of the classics of medical literature, *A Treatise of the Scurvy.* What was clear to Lind, and is commonplace to us, was not so readily accepted by the naval bureaucracy of his day. It took over forty years for the

British Admiralty to adopt Lind's simple prophylactic daily dose of one ounce of lemon juice per man. The official order came through in 1795, just a year after Lind's death. It has been estimated that this 42-year delay cost the Royal Navy 100,000 casualties to scurvy.

This simple regimen wiped out scurvy in the naval forces of England, and it became their secret weapon for maintaining their mastery of the seas. There is no doubt that this simple ration of lemon juice was of far greater importance to the Royal Navy of the eighteenth and nineteenth centuries than all the improvements in speed, firepower, armor, and seaworthiness. Naval officers of the time asserted that it was equivalent to doubling the fighting force of the navy. Previously, because of the ravages of scurvy, the seagoing fleets had to be relieved every ten weeks by a freshly manned fleet of equal strength so that the scorbutic seamen could be brought home for rehabilitation. The impact of our elusive molecule on history has never been adequately evaluated. In this case Lind did as much as Nelson to break the power of Napoleon. The English vessels were able to maintain continuous blockade duties, laying off the coast of France for months at a time without the necessity of relieving the men. Were it not for Lind, the flat-bottomed invasion barges assembled by Napoleon may well have crossed the English Channel.

6

THE NINETEENTH AND EARLY TWENTIETH CENTURIES

One would imagine that Lind's clear-cut clinical demonstration and the experiences of the Royal Navy in wiping out the disease would have pointed the way toward banishing this disease completely. However, it takes much more than logic and clear-cut demonstrations to overcome the inertia and dogma of established thought. The forty-two years that it took the British Admiralty to adopt Lind's recommendations may seem unduly long, even for a stolid bureaucracy, but this may be a speed record compared with other agencies. The British Board of Trade took 112 years—until 1865—before similar precautions were adopted for the British merchant marine. There are records of seamen on the merchant vessels succumbing to scurvy even while delivering lemons to the ships of the Royal Navy. Over 30,000 cases of scurvy were reported in the American Civil War and it took the U.S. Army until 1895 to adopt antiscorbutic rations.

The saga of scurvy continues, with its incredible toll in human lives and suffering, up to the present day. In the nineteenth century, 104 land epidemics have been tabulated. And the twentieth century has had plenty of trouble with the disease, not only as a result of the World Wars but, in civil populations, as a result of ignorance and improper use of food.

In the latter part of the nineteenth century, Barlow's disease became prevalent, and it was recognized as infantile scurvy. It appeared at the time when artificial feeding of babies was becoming popular, and took the name of the doctor who described the disease in 1883. Actually, the disease was first described in 1650, but it was confused with rickets until Barlow's clear differentiation. There were so many cases that it was also known as Mueller's or Cheadle's disease. Breast-fed babies did not appear to get the disease, but those fed with boiled and heated cow's milk or with cereal substitutes did. It is an intensively painful disease and results in stunted growth and delayed development. The disease persists to the present day and is amenable to the same preventive and curative measures as adult scurvy—the speck of ascorbic acid contained in fresh fruits and vegetables. Here again the lesson had to be relearned, the hard way, with babies put in the same class as seamen.

Scurvy and its treatment has had many ups and downs during the long history of man, and one series of events in the nineteenth century raised some mistrust in the prophylactic powers of fresh fruits. This is another example of the kind of mistaken conclusions based on confusion, incomplete observations, and improper interpretations which has cursed the history of scurvy. At the time this took place all knowledge of scurvy was completely empirical; there was no experimental or quantitative data because there were no experimental animals known that could be given scurvy. We did not know any more than Lind knew a hundred years before.

The English used the term "lime" indiscriminately for both lemons and limes. In 1850, for political and economic reasons they substituted the West Indian lime for the traditional Mediterranean lemon used by the Royal Navy since 1795. We now know that the Mediterranean lemon is a good source of our elusive molecule, while the West Indian lime is not. In 1875 the Admiralty supplied a large amount of West Indian lime juice to Sir George Nare's expedition to discover the North Pole. An epidemic of scurvy broke out and ruined the expedition. A commission was appointed to inquire into the cause of the disaster but could arrive at no satisfactory conclusion. It was even more perplexing because a previous Arctic expedition in 1850 (the date is important because lemons were used) had spent two years of great hardships, but without scurvy. It took until 1919 to finally resolve the cause of this debacle; in the meantime, however, this incident provoked a general and indiscriminate distrust of antiscorbutics—especially among Polar explorers. On the Jackson-Harmsworth expedition of 1894–1897, a party carrying no lime juice, but eating large amounts of fresh bear meat, remained in good health. The crew left on the ship, taking their daily lime juice and subsisting on canned and salted meat, came down with scurvy. This led to the theory that scurvy was caused by tainted meat. Thus, in 1913, the Antarctic explorer, Captain Scott, and his companions suffered miserable deaths because their expedition was provisioned on the basis of the tainted meat theory and carried no antiscorbutics.

Because of the lack of accurate knowledge concerning our elusive molecule, many other odd theories on scurvy were proposed, some as late as the 1910s when we should have known better. One theory claimed that scurvy was due to an "acid intoxication" of the blood, another that it was a bacterial autointoxication, and, as late as 1916, someone "discovered" its bacterial origin. Probably the crowning nonsense was put forward in 1918, when it was claimed that constipation was the cause of scurvy. After World War I, two German doctors who had been assigned to care for Russian prisoners of war came up with the novel idea that scurvy was transmitted by vermin; apparently the Russians had both.

Aside from these blunders, the nineteenth century saw many great advances in the sciences. The germ theory of disease was established after much initial resistance from the medical dogma of the time. And progress was made in the scientific study of nutrition. A brief historical review of the science of nutrition will provide the reader with some background to better understand the theme of this book.

In the early years of the nineteenth century, experiments were conducted in which animals were fed purified diets of the then known food constituents: fats, carbohydrates, and proteins. But the animals did not thrive. Not only did they not grow well but they also developed an opacity of the cornea of the eye (which we now know is due to a vitamin A deficiency). Later in the century, in

1857 in Africa, Dr. Livingstone noted a similar eye condition in poorly fed natives. Later, about 1865, similar observations were made of slaves on South American sugar plantations. The condition was attributed to some toxic constituent in their monotonous diet rather than the lack of some element. Most of the investigators in the growing science of nutrition concentrated on learning the basic facts about calories and the utilization of fats, carbohydrates, and proteins in the diet. Why a purified diet, adequate in these elements, would not support life, long remained a mystery.

In the latter decades of the nineteenth century and early in the twentieth century, many important observations were made which helped unravel this mystery. The Japanese Tahaki showed that the disease beriberi, then afflicting 25 to 40 percent of the Imperial Japanese Fleet, could be prevented by adding meat, vegetables, and condensed milk to the customary diet of rice and fish. He missed the significance of his results because he believed the improvement was due to a higher calorie intake comparable to that of the German and British navies. In 1897, the Dutchman Eijkman, working in Batavia, was able to produce beriberi in chickens by feeding them polished rice (rice from which the husk coating is removed) and was able to cure the birds by giving them extracts of the husk or polishings. But he did not interpret his experiments correctly either. He thought that the polished rice contained a poison and the polishings contained a natural antidote. Four years later another Dutchman correctly interpreted these experiments, suggesting that beriberi in birds and men is caused by the lack of some vital substance in the polished rice that is present in the rice bran.

In 1905 and 1906, Pekelharing in Holland and Hopkins at Cambridge, England, repeated the old experiment of feeding rats and mice on purified diets and again found that they failed to grow and died young. But they went one step further and found that adding small amounts of milk, not exceeding four percent of the diet, allowed the animals to grow and live. Both investigators realized that there was something present in natural foods that is vitally important to good nutrition. The concept of deficiency diseases (the idea that a disease could be caused by something lacking in the diet) was dawning.

Two Norwegian workers, Holst and Fröhlich, in 1907, were also investigating beriberi, which was common among the sailors of the Norwegian fishing fleet. They were able to produce the disease in

chickens and pigeons but they wanted another experimental animal, a mammal, to work with. They chose the guinea pig, and a
fortunate choice it was for man and the science of nutrition. After
feeding the guinea pigs the beriberi-inducing diets, they found that
the guinea pigs rapidly came down with scurvy instead. This was a
startling discovery, because up to this point it was believed that
man was the only animal that could contract scurvy. This was also
a very valuable and practical contribution because now an experimental animal was available that could be used for all sorts of
exact and quantitative studies of scurvy. It also showed that there
was something very similar and unique about the physiology of the
guinea pig and man. This simple observation was the greatest
advance in the study of scurvy since the experiments of Lind in the
1740s. This discovery could have been made twelve years earlier
had Theobald Smith, the famous American pathologist, realized the
importance of his observation that guinea pigs fed a diet of oats
developed a hemorrhagic disease. But he failed to relate the bleeding of his guinea pigs with human scurvy.

There were many brilliant workers in the field of nutrition, but
we need only mention one other in the thread of occurrences that
led to the present misconceptions regarding our elusive molecule.
Casimir Funk, working in the Lister Institute, prepared a highly
concentrated rice-bran extract for the treatment of beriberi and
designated the curative substance in this extract as a "vitamine." In
1912–1913 he published his then radical theory that beriberi,
scurvy, and pellagra and possibly rickets and sprue were all "deficiency diseases," caused by the lack of some important specific trace
factor in the diet. Subsequent work divided these factors into three
groups: vitamin A, the fat-soluble antiophthalmic factor; vitamin
B, the water-soluble antineuritic substance; and vitamin C, the
water-soluble antiscorbutic material. It was not known for many
years whether each vitamin represented a single substance or
many. Vitamin B was later found to consist of a group of chemically diverse compounds, while both vitamin A and vitamin C were
single substances. Time added more "letters" to the vitamin alpha-
bet. Eventually the different vitamins were isolated, purified, and
their chemical structures determined and finally synthesized; but
this took many years.

In the early decades of the twentieth century, ascorbic acid was
still unknown. The sum total of our knowledge was about equal to
Lind's, but great changes were in store.

7

FINDING THE ELUSIVE MOLECULE

In 1907, with the discovery that guinea pigs were also susceptible to scurvy, experimental work heretofore impossible could be
conducted in the study of the disease. Foods could be assayed to
determine the amount of antiscorbutic substance they contained. The
general properties of our elusive molecule could be studied by
using various chemical treatments on the antiscorbutic extracts and
following them with animal assays to learn why the molecule was
so elusive and sensitive.

The bulk of the experiments on scurvy in the early years of the
twentieth century was carried out by nutritionists who had con-
trived the vitamin hypothesis and the concept of deficiency diseases. They had already taken scurvy under their wing as a typical
dietary deficiency disease. They had even named its cause and
cure, vitamin C, without knowing anything more definite than the
fact that it was some vague factor in fresh vegetables and fruits.

While the nutritionists were busy with their rats, mice, guinea
pigs, and vitamin theories, another important event took place in

medicine. We will mention it briefly here because it happened at about this time, and we will come back to it later to explain its significance to ascorbic acid and scurvy.

In 1908, the great English physician, Sir Archibald Garrod, presented a remarkable series of papers in which he set forth new ideas on inherited metabolic diseases, or as he stated it, "inborn errors of metabolism." These are diseases due to the inherited lack of certain enzymes. This lack may cause a variety of genetic diseases depending upon which particular enzyme is missing. The fatality of these diseases depends upon the importance of the biochemical process controlled by the missing enzyme. It may vary from relatively benign to rapidly fatal conditions. This was a revolutionary concept for those days—a disease caused by a biochemical defect in one's inheritance.

Now getting back to the main thread of our story, the nutritionists continued their work with their new-found experimental animals and in the next decades uncovered more information about our elusive molecule.

To study the chemistry of a substance such as ascorbic acid, it is necessary to concentrate it from the natural extracts, to isolate it in pure form, to crystallize it, and to recrystallize it to make sure it is just one single chemical compound. Only then can it be identified chemically, and its molecular structure determined. Once the structure of the compound is known, it is relatively easy to find ways to synthesize it. Comparison of the synthetic material with those of the original crystals will either confirm or deny whether the chemist's tests and reasoning were correct.

In the early 1920s scientists began concentrating the vitamin C factor and studying its behavior under various chemical treatments by means of quantitative animal assays. It was a long drawn-out procedure but it was gradually becoming clear why the molecule vanished so easily. The real tests, however, had to await its isolation and crystallization in pure form.

As scientists approached the home stretch of their search, the pace quickened and attracted more workers. There was a group at the Lister Institute in England and another in the United States; a Russian directed a group in France and later other groups formed. History has a way of playing tricks on the course of events. In the years before our elusive molecule was finally pinned down, there were a few close calls in the attempts to isolate it in pure form which, for one reason or another, were never successful. In the early 1920s a student worker at the University of Wisconsin, studying the biochemistry of oats, isolated a crude crystalline fraction which may have been our elusive material. The work was carried no further because the dean refused a research grant of a few hundred dollars which was required to pay for animal assays of these crude crystals. In 1925, two U.S. Army workers at Edgewood Arsenal were on the verge of obtaining crystals of the antiscorbutic substance when they were transferred to different stations; their work was never completed. Bezssonov, the Russian worker in France, may have isolated antiscorbutic crystals from cabbage juice in 1925, but for some unknown reason these crystals were never thoroughly investigated.

In 1928, Albert Szent-Gyorgyi, working at Cambridge, England, on a biochemical problem unrelated to scurvy or vitamin C, reported that he had isolated crystals of a new sugarlike substance with very unusual chemical properties from the adrenal gland of the ox. He called the substance "hexuronic acid." Similar crystals were also isolated from oranges and cabbages. While these crystals were isolated in connection with another biochemical problem, Szent-Gyorgyi noted their similarity to the chemical reactions of vitamin C and suspected there was some connection. He made arrangements to have the crystals tested by animal assay but before he could obtain enough crystals he left England and the matter was left in abeyance. It was not until 1931, after he had resettled in Hungary, that he was able to pick up the threads and carry out the necessary tests which proved hexuronic acid to be vitamin C. In that year, a student of Hungarian descent, J. L. Svirbely, who had worked with the American team of vitamin C researchers at the University of Pittsburgh under Charles Glenn King, returned to Hungary and joined forces with Szent-Gyorgyi to work on the problem. The years 1932 and 1933 were very fruitful and saw many published reports by American, Hungarian, English, and other workers. All this research showed that hexuronic acid was indeed our elusive molecule, and it was soon renamed "ascorbic acid."

With the pure crystals of ascorbic acid available, its chemical structure was quickly determined and methods for its synthetic production from the sugars were devised. The development of these syntheses permitted unlimited production of ascorbic acid at a low price and provided a practical solution to a problem that had always beleaguered man—but of which he was still unaware.

Thus our elusive molecule was finally pinned down and revealed. The search had ended. The importance of this work was recognized in 1937 by the award of two Nobel Prizes: one to Szent-Gyorgyi for his biochemical discoveries and the other to the English chemist, Sir Walter Haworth, for his research on the chemical structure and synthesis of ascorbic acid.

8

THE GENETIC APPROACH

Although the search for our elusive molecule has ended, our story has not. Actually, the means for ascorbic acid's unlimited synthetic production provide us with a second beginning. We shall now see how the subsequent investigations of the following forty years got off to a wrong start which hindered our understanding of this unique molecule and the thorough exploitation of its vast therapeutic potentialities. To better understand the circumstances of this paradoxical situation, we will try to look into the mental climate of the most advanced investigators in this field in the early 1930s. A reader of the previous historical chapters would know vastly more about ascorbic acid and its place in human evolution than anyone in that era. The mechanisms of the natural synthesis of ascorbic acid by plants and animals were still unknown and their genetic significance was not even a gleam in any researcher's eye. The important enzyme L-gulonolactone oxidase was awaiting discovery in the far distant future and the importance of this and related enzyme systems were not even suspected. All the investigators had been brought up on the dogmatic tenets of the then thirty-year-old vitamin-C theory. Scurvy was an avitaminosis (a dietary deficiency disease) and this nutritional disturbance could be prevented or cured by ingesting minute amounts of this trace nutrient in the diet. Thus vitamin C was considered a trace food constituent found in certain foodstuffs and was not even remotely associated with the idea that it might have been a product of man's original metabolism.

In the early and mid-1930s the status of scurvy had changed little from the time of Lind in 1753 when it was considered a food-related disease, except that 20 years earlier someone had called the unknown substance a "vitamine." As time rolled on and more facts were gathered, it seemed that "vitamin C" was not behaving like a typical vitamin. For nearly all animals it was not even a "vitamin" because of its widespread manufacture in their own bodies; they never got scurvy no matter how little vitamin C was in their food. Out of the thousands of different animals existing in Nature only three (man, monkeys, and guinea pigs) were known to need vitamin C in their foodstuffs. The effective dosages of vitamin C were also considerably higher than those for the other known vitamins. As the chemical and enzymatic mechanisms of how plants and animals make their own vitamin C became known, the terms "vitamin C" and "ascorbic acid" became more and more synonymous. In the field of biochemical genetics, great advances were being made in understanding the mechanisms of heredity. A vast amount of clinical work was reported on the use of ascorbic acid in the treatment of all known diseases, much without spectacular success except in the case of scurvy. These developments and others, covering a quarter of a century, were instrumental in shaping the author's genetic concepts of the human need for ascorbic acid. The vitamin C hypothesis never attempted to explain *why* we were susceptible to scurvy, only how we got it. This hypothesis no longer served the new accumulation of facts, and clearly a new approach was required. However, up until 1966, the vitamin C hypothesis was an unquestioned part of published medical dogma.

For the development of these new concepts we have to return to Sir Archibald Garrod, mentioned in the last chapter, who in 1908 introduced the concept of the inherited enzyme disease into medicine. At the time, this was a revolutionary way of explaining the cause of disease in man. These genetic diseases are caused by the inherited lack or inactivity of a certain specific enzyme. The inability of the enzyme to function normally prevents the body from carrying out the biochemical process involved. This may cause toxic by-products to accumulate or abnormal biochemical pathways to develop which bring on the symptoms of the genetic disease. As mentioned earlier, the diseases range from the relatively harmless to those that are rapidly fatal. The reader will remember that the body contains thousands of enzymes for carrying out the living process and the absence of any one can bring on an "inborn error of metabolism." Since each of the body's enzymes is synthesized from a single gene in the chromosome, a slight mutation of the gene can cause the loss of an enzyme and thus cause a genetic disease.

Sir Archibald, in his original 1908 papers, described four genetic diseases, but the list has now grown and new ones are constantly being reported. He reported on albinism, alkaptonuria, cystinuria, and pentosuria, all due to the lack of a particular enzyme in the afflicted individual's biochemical inheritance. Albinism, a relatively harmless condition, is due to the lack of an enzyme used in the production of the black skin pigment, melanin. Alkaptonuria and cystinuria are both diseases of protein metabolism in which the missing enzyme causes an accumulation of intermediate protein digestion products, which causes changes in the urine and other parts of the body. Alkaptonuria is relatively benign until later in life when it produces a severe type of arthritic condition. Cystinuria induces the formation of kidney and bladder stones, while the relatively rare and harmless pentosuria causes pentose, a sugar, to appear in the urine and may be confused with diabetes.

Like many other great discoveries in medicine, Garrod's work was almost ignored for a generation. In fact, an examination of the major genetics textbooks in use in 1940 fails to reveal any mention of alkaptonuria, described by Garrod thirty-two years earlier. Time has corrected this oversight and the importance of Garrod's pioneering work is now acknowledged by all.

Two other more recent genetic diseases, now much in the news, will be briefly mentioned: galactosemia, which afflicts infants, is caused by a missing enzyme, galactose-1-phosphate-uridyl-transferase, (all enzyme names end with "ase") that prevents babies from properly digesting the sugar in milk. Unless they are promptly taken off a milk diet, they will sicken and may die. Those that survive will be stunted in growth, may develop cataracts, and may be mentally retarded. The other genetic disease, phenyl-ketonuria (or PKU), is another disease of infants and is caused by the inherited lack of the enzyme, phenylalanine hydroxylase, pro-ducing a profound disturbance of protein digestion. Unless the vic-tims are placed on special low-protein diets, irreversible brain damage can occur as well as mental retardation and other nervous disorders.

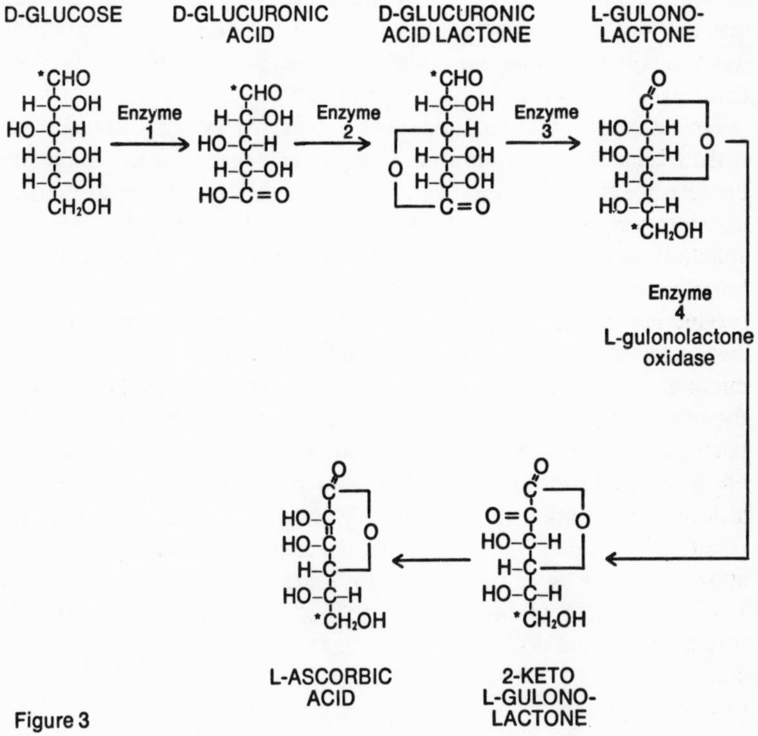

Figure 3

Now back to ascorbic acid. In mammals, ascorbic acid is pro-duced in the liver from blood glucose by the stepwise reactions shown in Figure 3. Each step, except the last, is controlled by a specific enzyme. In the last step, the 2-keto-L-gulonolactone, once formed, is automatically converted into ascorbic acid. No enzyme is required. On the right side of the diagram, the step of transforming L-gulonolactone into 2-keto-L-gulonolactone is catalyzed by the enzyme L-gulonolactone oxidase. This is the critical enzyme for humans who, because they carry a defective gene, cannot produce an active enzyme. This is the gene that mutated in a primate ancestor of ours millions of years ago. It is this step that is blocked in man and prevents him from producing large amounts of ascorbic acid from glucose in the liver.

Here we have the classic conditions for a genetic, missing-enzyme disease, and yet for years these simple facts have been ignored and scurvy has continued to be regarded as an avitamin-osis. In 1966, this author published the paper "On the Genetic Etiology of Scurvy," in which the history and pertinent facts were reviewed and it was pointed out that in scurvy we were dealing with a genetic, liver-enzyme disease and not simply a dietary disturbance. Since it is the prerogative of the discoverer to name a new disease, the author called it "hypoascorbemia" because low levels of ascorbic acid in the blood are characteristic of this disease.

This genetic approach now provides a natural rationale for the use of large amounts of ascorbic acid which served so well in the survival of the mammals in the course of evolution. Its implications for health and well-being are vast because it furnishes the basis for the new unexplored fields of preventive medicine and therapeutics (megascorbic prophylaxis and megascorbic therapy). It is hoped that the publication of these new ways of using ascorbic acid will stimulate the flood of research similar to that which occurred when ascorbic acid was discovered in the early 1930s. Let us see how long it will take to break down the "vitamin-barriers" of current orthodox medical dogma.

9

SOME EFFECTS OF
ASCORBIC ACID

At this point it is best to discuss briefly some of the effects of ascorbic acid on various important bodily functions. This will give the reader a better insight and background for the later chapters. Ascorbic acid is involved in so many vital biochemical processes and is so important in daily living that, after forty years of research, we still have no clear idea of all the ways in which it works.

Throughout the evolution of the vertebrates, including the mammals, Nature has used ascorbic acid to maintain physiological homeostasis. In simple nontechnical terms, this means that when stressful situations arose which disturbed the biochemical equilibrium of the animal, ascorbic acid was produced in increased quantities to get things running normal again. The amount of ascorbic acid produced is related to the severity of the stresses and if enough was produced soon enough, then the animal was able to survive the bad biochemical effects of the stresses. If, however, the enzyme system for producing ascorbic acid was overwhelmed or poisoned by the stresses and too little ascorbic acid was produced, then the animal succumbed. Man, unable to produce his own ascorbic acid, could not take advantage of this natural protective process. Instead, stresses only further depleted his low stores of this vital metabolite. Now he can easily duplicate this time-tested defensive mechanism by reaching for the bottle of ascorbic acid and swallowing additional quantities whenever he is subjected to biochemical stresses. In duplicating this normal process for combating stresses, man has one great advantage over the other mammals—he can get an unlimited supply of ascorbic acid without being dependent upon an enzyme system which may not produce enough, quickly enough. All man needs to know is how much to take.

One of the outstanding attributes of ascorbic acid is its lack of toxicity even when given in large doses over long periods of time. This has been recognized since the 1930s, and ascorbic acid can be rated as one of the least toxic substances known of comparable physiological activity. It can be administered in huge doses, intravenously, without registering any serious side effects. Because of human variability and because the human organism has been exposed to such low levels of this essential substance for so long, some usually transient side effects may occur in a small percentage of hypersensitive individuals. This may be evidenced as diarrhea or rashes which clear up on lowering the dosage. In many cases it is possible to avoid these reactions by building up to the desired dosage gradually, which permits the body to become accustomed to these essentially normal mammalian levels. Taking the ascorbic acid with food or before meals often helps.

Chemically, ascorbic acid is a rather simple carbohydrate related to the blood sugar, glucose (see Figure 1, page 9). Unlike glucose, it contains an unusual, highly reactive combination of molecules called the "ene-diol group." The presence of this group confers upon the ascorbic acid molecule certain unique biochemical characteristics which may explain its vital importance in the living process. It transforms a relatively inactive sugar into a highly reactive, labile, and reversible carbohydrate derivative which readily donates or accepts electrons from its surrounding medium. This is known technically as an "oxidation-reduction system."

On a molecular basis, the whole living process is nothing more than an orderly flow and transfer of electrons. Therefore, having an abundance of a substance like ascorbic acid present in living matter makes this orderly flow and transfer of electrons proceed with greater ease and facility. It acts substantially like an oil for the machinery of life. This was discovered by Nature billions of years ago. Recent work indicates that this oxidation-reduction system can form even more active free radicals which may explain some of its unusual biological effects.

There are no large storage depots for ascorbic acid in the body and any excess is rapidly excreted. When saturated, the whole body may only contain 5 grams. This means that the body requires a continuous supply to replenish losses and depletions. The livers of nearly all mammals are constantly making and pouring ascorbic acid into their bloodstreams, but man's liver is unable to do this. He needs a constant, large, outside supply to make up for this genetic defect. When the different organs and tissues are analyzed, it is found that ascorbic acid concentrates in the organs and tissues with high metabolic activity: the adrenal cortex, the pituitary gland, the brain, the ovaries, the eyes, and other vital tissues. Any form of biochemical stress or physical trauma will cause a precipitous drop in the ascorbic acid levels of the body in general, or locally in the affected organs or tissues. In animals biochemically equipped to produce their own ascorbic acid, any stressful situation causes them to synthesize more and greater amounts to replace that destroyed or utilized in combating the stresses.

One of the most important biochemical functions of ascorbic acid in the body's chemistry is the synthesis, formation, and maintenance of a proteinlike substance called collagen. Collagen cannot be formed without ascorbic acid, which is absolutely essential to collagen production by the body. Collagen is the body's most important structural substance. It is the ground substance, or cement, that supports and holds the tissues and organs together. It is the substance in the bones that provides the toughness and flexibility and prevents brittleness. Without it the body would just disintegrate or dissolve away. It comprises about one-third of the body's total weight of protein and is the most extensive tissue system. It is the substance that strengthens the arteries and veins, supports the muscles, toughens the ligaments and bones, supplies the scar tissue for healing wounds and keeps the youthful skin tissues soft, firm, supple and wrinkle-free. When ascorbic acid is lacking, it is the disturbance in collagen formation that causes the fearful effects of scurvy—the brittle bones that fracture on the slightest impact, the weakened arteries that rupture and hemorrhage, the incapacitating muscle weakness, the affected joints that are too painful to move, the teeth that fall out, and the wounds and sores that never heal. Suboptimal amounts of ascorbic acid over prolonged periods during the early and middle years, by its effect of producing poor quality collagen, may be the factor in later life that causes the high incidence of arthritis and joint diseases, broken hips, the heart and vascular diseases that cause sudden death, and the strokes that bring on senility. Collagen is intimately connected with the entire aging process.

Ascorbic acid has a marked activating effect on many bodily enzymes and makes the processes controlled by these enzymes proceed at a more favorable rate. It is very important in nutrition, the digestion of food, and the biochemistry of the body's utilization of carbohydrates, proteins, and fats. In carbohydrate metabolism it has a pronounced activating effect on insulin. It is essential to the proper functioning of the nervous system. Brain chemistry is dependent on the maintenance of proper levels of ascorbic acid and high levels are essential in treating nervous and mental disorders, as we shall see in a later chapter.

Ascorbic acid is a potent detoxicant which counteracts and neutralizes the harmful effects of many poisons in the body. It will combat various inorganic poisons, such as mercury and arsenic, and it neutralizes the bad reactions of many organic poisons, drugs, and bacterial and animal toxins. Ascorbic acid detoxifies carbon monoxide, sulfur dioxide, and carcinogens, so it is the only immediate protection we have against the bad effects of air pollution and smoking. It has also been shown that ascorbic acid increases the therapeutic effect of different drugs and medicines by making them more effective. Thus, less of a drug is required if it is taken in combination with large amounts of ascorbic acid. Diabetics could reduce their insulin requirements if this were practiced. Even an aspirin should be accompanied by a large dose of ascorbic acid to heighten its analgesic effect and lessen its toxic action on the body.

Ascorbic acid in large doses is a good nontoxic diuretic. A diuretic is a substance that stimulates the excretion of urine. Thus, ascorbic acid at proper dosage levels will drain waterlogged tissues and reduce accumulated water in the body in heart and kidney diseases.

The antiseptic and bactericidal qualities of ascorbic acid have long been known. At relatively low levels it will inhibit the growth of bacteria and at slightly higher amounts it will kill them. The bacteria causing tuberculosis is particularly sensitive to the lethal action of ascorbic acid.

One of the body's defenses against bacterial infections is the mobilization of white blood cells into the affected tissues. The white blood cells then devour and digest the invading bacteria. This process is known as phagocytosis and is controlled by ascorbic acid. The number of bacteria that each white blood cell digests is directly related to the ascorbic acid content of the blood. This is one of the reasons why a lack of ascorbic acid in the body produces lowered resistance to infectious diseases.

Ascorbic acid is also a potent and nonspecific virucide. It has the power to inactivate and destroy the infectivity of a wide variety of disease-producing viruses including poliomyelitis, herpes, vaccinia, foot-and-mouth disease, and rabies. It only does this, however, at relatively high doses, not at "vitamin" levels.

There is a relationship between ascorbic acid and the production and maintenance in the body of the adrenal cortical hormones. The adrenal gland, where this hormone is produced, also happens to be the tissue where the highest concentration of ascorbic acid is found.

In 1969 it was reported that laboratory tests conducted at the National Cancer Institute showed that ascorbic acid was lethal to certain cancer cells and harmless to normal tissue. This might be the long awaited breakthrough in cancer therapy. Intensive study and research should immediately be concentrated to investigate these possibilities.

This has been a brief and incomplete summary of ascorbic acid's many biochemical functions and of its vital importance in keeping the body in good operating condition. Even this incomplete review should not only give the reader an idea of the many important functions of ascorbic acid, but also leave the very distinct impression that ascorbic acid can be of much greater use to man than as a mere prevention of clinical symptoms of scurvy.

10

"CORRECTING" NATURE

No one would have any difficulty recognizing the violent, extreme symptoms of totally "uncorrected" hypoascorbemia—the clinical scurvy; but the milder forms, from which most people suffer, are difficult to detect. Chronic hypoascorbemia, or as it was previously called, "subclinical scurvy," is relatively symptom-free and can only be diagnosed by clinical or chemical testing, or by difficult long-term observations. Acute scurvy in the well-developed nations is, nowadays, not a common disease for two reasons. First, the daily amounts of ascorbic acid needed to protect against the symptoms of clinical scurvy are very small and, second, the improvements in food preservation and distribution make it easy to obtain these small amounts in foods available the year round. This is not the case, however, for chronic hypoascorbemia. Anyone who depends solely on foodstuffs for ascorbic acid cannot expect "full correction" of hypoascorbemia. The more stress that such an individual is under, the higher would be the deficit. It is the lack of recognition of the distinction between acute scurvy and chronic hypoascorbemia, and the narrow aims of the "vitamin" theory, that have given a false sense of security, for the past sixty years, as to the adequacy of foodstuffs to fully supply the body's needs for ascorbic acid.

Hypoascorbemia can be "corrected" by supplying the individual with ascorbic acid in the amounts the liver would be making and supplying to the body if the enzyme were not missing. How, then, can we determine the amounts of ascorbic acid the human liver would be producing by an enzyme that is not there? The solution to this question may not be as difficult as it may seem at first glance. If the requirements for ascorbic acid in man are assumed to be similar to those of other, closely related mammals, then, by measuring the amounts of ascorbic acid produced by other mammals, we should be able to get a pretty good estimate of what man would be making, had he the complete synthetic enzyme system.

When we look for this very important data in the literature, it is amazing how little we find. The only information available is on the rat. No one has bothered to determine the amounts of ascorbic acid the larger mammals such as the pig, dog, or horse are capable of producing.

Clearly, a great deal more research is required to determine the extent of ascorbic acid synthesis by different mammals so that a more accurate estimate of man's needs can be calculated. Until this work is completed, we are forced to rely on the figures presently available for the rat.

From these available figures, "full correction" of hypoascorbemia in a 70-kilogram adult human is estimated to require a daily intake of 2,000 to 4,000 milligrams (2.0 to 4.0 grams) of ascorbic acid, under conditions of little or no stress. Under conditions of stress, the data indicates an increase to about 15,000 milligrams (15.0 grams) per day. Under very severe stresses, even more may be required.

Biochemical stress covers a wide range of conditions, among which may be mentioned: bacterial and viral infections, physical trauma, injuries and burns, exposure to heat, cold, or noxious fumes, ingestion of drugs and poisons, air pollution and smoking, surgery, worry, aging, and many others.

Ascorbic acid is rapidly absorbed from the digestive tract so that "full correction" can be established by giving it, preferably in solution, in several oral doses during the day. This is easily and pleasantly accomplished by dissolving a one-half level teaspoonful of ascorbic acid powder (1,500 milligrams or 1.5 grams) in a half glass of fruit or tomato juice or in about two ounces of water sweetened to taste. A dose in the morning and another at night and possibly one midday should establish "full correction" under conditions of no unusual stresses. This basic regimen for "normal" individuals should be the subject matter of extensive long-term clinical trials by statistically sufficient numbers of subjects of different age groups, to determine the long-range effects of these "corrective" dosage levels of ascorbic acid on their well-being, disease resistance, disease morbidity, the inhibiting effects on aging, and the possible lengthening of the human life span. The medical authorities supervising this proposed research, if and when it is conducted, should be convinced of its safety because: 1. these are normal mammalian ascorbic acid levels, 2. ascorbic acid virtually lacks toxicity, and 3. countless generations of monkeys have been raised using these ascorbic acid levels throughout their lives with the diet recommended by the National Research Council of the National Academy of Sciences.

Under conditions of biochemical stress, the frequency and size of the doses are increased depending upon severity of the stress. Amounts over 100 grams (100,000 milligrams) per day have been suggested for the therapy of acute viral infections. Clinical trials and dosages for the therapy of specific conditions will be discussed in later chapters.

The known lack of toxicity of ascorbic acid would indicate that no general serious side effects or toxic reactions would be incident to these "full correction" regimens. One mild discomfort that has been noted is diarrhea in individuals whose digestive tract is hypersensitive to the cathartic effect of fruit acids. The diarrhea stopped when the dosage was reduced and no other sequela resulted. Administration by injection has been used, but the oral route is so much simpler and pleasanter that intravenous doses may be reserved for cases where the oral route is not feasible or very severe stresses require heroic measures for building high blood levels of ascorbic acid quickly under medical supervision.

If gastric distress is encountered due to the acidity of the ascorbic acid, partial neutralization with small amounts of sodium bicarbonate or the use of sodium ascorbate instead of ascorbic acid will overcome this (see Chapter 21).

"Full correction" of this genetic disease has only been possible since the late 1930s when the synthetic production of ascorbic acid made it available in unlimited quantities at a low enough price. This "correction" could never be established by dependence upon ascorbic acid-containing foodstuffs because it is just physically impossible to ingest the large volumes of foods required to give the necessary dosage levels.

Actually this "full correction" concept merely attempts to duplicate in man a normal physiological process which is taking place all the time in other mammals, and that is to supply ascorbic acid in amounts in accordance with the needs.

The National Research Council of the National Academy of Sciences publishes reports from their Food and Nutrition Board and their Committee on Animal Nutrition. These are published as bulletins, available to the public, and they are the authoritative, last word on the nutrient requirements of humans and animals. The Food and Nutrition Board's bulletin on human needs is entitled "Recommended Dietary Allowances" (Seventh Revised Edition, 1968) and gives the recommended daily allowance for an adult human for ascorbic acid as 60 milligrams per day (about one milligram per kilogram of body weight). From the Committee on Animal Nutrition's "Nutrient Requirements of Laboratory Animals" (1962) we find some startling figures. The recommended diet for the monkey—our closest mammalian relative—is 55 milligrams of ascorbic acid per kilogram of body weight or 3,830 milligrams of ascorbic acid per day for the average adult human. The daily amount suggested as adequate for the guinea pig varies depending upon which of two diets is selected and ranges from 42 to 167 milligrams per kilogram of body weight (based on a 300-gram guinea pig). This amounts to 2,920 milligrams to 11,650 milligrams per day for the average adult human.

In summary, on an equivalent body weight basis the daily intake of ascorbic acid recommended by the National Research Council for humans is 60 milligrams; for monkeys, 3,830 milligrams; and for guinea pigs, 2,920 to 11,650 milligrams. It is noteworthy that the figure for the monkeys is similar to our estimate of the daily amount that would be produced in the human liver if the final essential enzyme were not missing. There is a 55-fold difference between the amount recommended for man and that given for monkeys; and the guinea pigs have a 42- to 167-fold advantage over man. Are these agencies shortchanging the human population in favor of laboratory animals? The pressure groups that are continually complaining of how badly laboratory animals are being treated certainly would have no complaint on this score. It is time we had a pressure group to see that humans also receive enough ascorbic acid!

The author has not been alone in the belief that the present recommended levels of ascorbic acid may not be the optimal levels to fulfill all our requirements. In 1949, Geoffrey H. Bourne, now head of the Yerkes Regional Primate Research Center in Atlanta, Georgia, pointed out that an adult gorilla in the wild state consumes about 4.5 grams of ascorbic acid a day in his food. He also speculated that the recommended milligrams a day for humans might be wide of the mark and 1 or 2 grams a day might be the correct amount.

Dr. Albert Szent-Gyorgyi, who received the Nobel Prize in Medicine for his research on ascorbic acid, in a private communication to the author in 1965, stated that what he liked about the author's genetic concept is that it suggested "that the daily dosage of ascorbic acid in man should be much higher. I have always pleaded for such a higher dosage."

Dr. Frederick R. Klenner of Reidsville, North Carolina, who has had more actual clinical experience in megascorbic prophylaxis and megascorbic therapy in the past thirty years than anyone else in the world, routinely prescribes ten grams of ascorbic acid daily to his adult patients for the maintenance of good health. His daily dosage schedule for children is one gram of ascorbic acid per year of age up to ten years and ten grams daily thereafter (e.g., a four-year-old child would receive four grams daily).

Linus Pauling pioneered in the field of molecular diseases with the discovery, published in 1949, that sickle-cell anemia is due to slight, but very important, changes in the structure of the blood protein, hemoglobin. He has also been very active in developing concepts which indicate that we may have inadequate levels of various natural substances normally present in the body, and which can bring forth symptoms of disease. In 1967, in a communication to the Thirteenth International Convention on Vital Substances, Nutrition, and Diseases of Civilization, held in Luxembourg, Dr. Pauling described other molecular diseases and developed the concept of "orthomolecular therapy." Generally, orthomolecular therapy involves supplying vitamins, amino acids, or other natural bodily constituents which are at suboptimal levels by intakes of large amounts of the needed substance.

Dr. Pauling also described in this paper the application of ortho-molecular medicine to the treatment of mental disease by the provision of high levels of ascorbic acid and other vitamins as the preferred method of treatment. The subject of orthomolecular psy-chiatry was developed in further detail in a 1968 paper appearing in the April 19, 1968 issue of *Science*. In the book *Vitamin C and the Common Cold* published in 1970, Dr. Pauling devotes a chap-ter to orthomolecular medicine. The use of high levels of ascorbic acid in the prevention and treatment of the common cold is a practical application of the principles of orthomolecular medicine. Megascorbic prophylaxis and megascorbic therapy are, thus, branch-es of orthomolecular medicine.

In a paper presented by Dr. Pauling to the National Academy of Sciences and appearing in the December 15, 1970 issue of their *Proceedings,* calculations were made from the caloric and ascorbic acid content of raw plant foods. From this data, Dr. Pauling concluded that the optimum daily intake of ascorbic acid, for most human adults, is in the range of 2.3 grams to 9 grams. Because of the variation due to "biochemical individuality" the range of opti-mum intake for a large population may be as high as 250 milli-grams to 10,000 milligrams (10 grams) or more a day.

"Biochemical individuality" is a concept from the work of Pro-fessor Roger J. Williams at the University of Texas, which indi-cated that individuals vary over a considerable range in their need and use of metabolites and that a value based on a so-called average may be far off the mark.

Dr. Leon E. Rosenberg, Associate Professor of Pediatrics and Medicine at the Yale University School of Medicine, in discussing biochemical abnormalities due to hereditary defects, suggested dif-ferentiating between vitamin-deficiency diseases and vitamin-dependent diseases. The vitamin-dependent diseases are those which may require 10 to 1,000 times the "normal" daily require-ments for their successful treatment. Rosenberg's work was confined to vitamin-dependent genetic defects of the various B vitamins and vitamin D. He apparently has not worked with ascorbic acid.*

The interesting conclusion which can be drawn from: 1. the gorilla data of Bourne, 2. the evolutionary raw-plant food calcula-tions of Pauling, 3. the daily synthesis of ascorbic acid by the rat,

*This was reviewed in *Science News* of August 29, 1970, pages 157–158, and in the *Journal of the American Medical Association* of September 21, 1970, page 2001.

4. the dietary recommendations of the National Research Council for the good nutrition of monkeys, and 5. the actual human clinical data of Klenner, is that all of these point to an intake of several grams a day, rather than the sixty milligrams a day now regarded as adequate.

PART II
Pathways to Research

11

BREAKING THE "VITAMIN" BARRIER

The discovery of ascorbic acid and its identification as the anti-scorbutic substance vitamin C in 1933 literally launched thousands of medical research projects on practically every known disease and pathologic condition. Here was a newly discovered substance of extremely unusual medicinal properties with almost magical curative properties for scurvy. A person at death's door from scurvy could be miraculously returned to health in a few days with a few specks of ascorbic acid.

The number of medical research papers published and the variety of diseases covered in the flood of research triggered by this discovery were so great that five years later, in 1938, a contemporary author remarked, "So many papers have now been published on this subject that it is difficult to find a single ailment to which the human or animal body is prone that has not been investigated." In 1938 and again in 1939, over six hundred medical research papers on ascorbic acid were published throughout the world.

In reviewing this tremendous volume of medical literature, one is struck by the dominating influence that the nutritional and vitamin aspects of ascorbic acid had on most of these medical investigators. This was due to their thorough indoctrination in the vitamin C hypothesis. For them, the antiscorbutic substance could only be a vitamin, and scurvy was just a dietary irregularity. They also knew that the merest trace of ascorbic acid, a few milligrams a day, would serve as a curative dose for scurvy. Thus, when they tackled other diseases in the early 1930s, they used dosage levels found satisfactory for scurvy. While many of the therapeutic results indicated encouraging good effects, just as many showed a lack of notable success and even failures, and much confusion resulted. It is this low-dosage bias that throws grave doubts on the usefulness of the clinical results reported over the next several decades.

These early investigators also had practical reasons for using the low-dosage levels. In the early 1930s, ascorbic acid was a relatively rare and expensive commodity which was rationed by the early sources of supply. Investigators were limited by availability and could not have given bigger doses, even if they had wanted to. In the late 1930s, scarcity was no longer a problem since large-scale synthetic production was getting underway and there was a substantial drop in prices. But the low-dosage tests continued.

In those early days, therapeutic doses of 50 to 100 milligrams per day were considered "large" and by vitamin criteria they were. It is thoroughly disheartening, however, to go through the later literature and find in paper after paper, in spite of the early lack of success, the continued use of these low-dosage levels. These workers repeated and repeated the early mistake of using ineffective, small dosages. Hardly anyone was inspired to increase the dosages and test higher levels to see if they were more effective. This situation is even stranger when we remember that ascorbic acid is a substance with virtually no toxicity, so there was no danger from a substantial dosage increase. These workers were so imbued with the "vitamin" concepts that they could not conceive of giving a so-called vitamin at the dosage rate of many grams per day. This "vitamin" mental block prevented them from applying the common principle of pharmacology of adjusting the dosage level to get the effect desired. They thought of ascorbic acid as a "vitamin" and as a "vitamin" they expected miracles from trace amounts. What was needed was "medication," not "alimentation," but this simple fact escaped the majority of investigators.

Successful therapy with ascorbic acid was reported, but only in the work of the few investigators who used sufficiently high dosages of many grams per day. These rare individuals were the ones who provided the foundations of megascorbic therapy, which have to be more thoroughly extended and explored. The genetic disease concept now provides a clear and definite rationale for the use of these multigram doses.

One of the few clinical investigators who realized the importance of dosage levels in ascorbic acid therapy was Dr. F. R. Klenner, who, in the late 1940s and early 1950s, successfully pioneered the therapy of viral diseases with large daily doses of ascorbic acid. His remarkable and dramatic therapeutic results in diseases such as poliomyelitis, still largely ignored by medicine, will be discussed in the chapter on viral diseases, but let us read his views on the work preceding his studies.

A review of the literature in preparation of this paper, however, presented an almost unbelievable record of such studies. The years of labor in animal experimentations, the cost in human effort and in "grants" and the volumes written, make it difficult to understand how so many investigators could have failed in comprehending the one thing that would have given positive results a decade ago. This one thing was the size of the dose of vitamin C employed and the frequency of its administration. . . . No one would expect to relieve kidney colic with a five-grain aspirin tablet; by the same logic we cannot hope to destroy the virus organism with doses of vitamin C of 10 to 400 milligrams. The results which we have reported in virus diseases using vitamin C as the antibiotic may seem fantastic. These results, however, are no different from the results we see when administering the sulfa, or mold-derived drugs against many other kinds of infections. In the latter instances we expect and usually get forty-eight- to seventy-two-hour cures; it is laying no claim to miracle working, then, when we say that many virus infections can be cleared within a similar time limit [with ascorbic acid].*

This lone voice has been echoing, unheeded, through the maze of medical literature for nearly two decades, while the still-unsuccessful search for another anti-viral agent still goes on.

*These comments are contained in his 1949 paper entitled, "The Treatment of Poliomyelitis and Other Virus Diseases with Vitamin C."

The following chapters will briefly summarize the clinical experiences, as reported in the medical literature of the past forty years on ascorbic acid therapy of a wide variety of diseases. Provocative ideas and results will be pointed out and further lines of research will be suggested. The time has come to reassess this previous work with the new genetic concepts in mind, and to start long-term investigations of these inadequately explored areas. It will be necessary to break down the sixty-year-old vitamin C mental barriers that have impeded research thus far and to apply some logic to the protocols of clinical research. Ascorbic acid has been thoroughly tried at nutritional levels, over the years, without notable success. It is high time that megascorbic levels become the subject of clinical testing.

Before embarking on the large-scale clinical trials urged in later chapters, further information and additional tests should be conducted to resolve questions in three areas. First of all, the data on the estimated daily production of ascorbic acid in man is based on the results of tests on rats. It would be desirable to obtain additional data on the daily synthesis of ascorbic acid in the larger mammals under varying conditions of stress. In this way we could get a closer estimate of what man would be producing in his liver, if he did not carry the defective gene for L-gulonolactone oxidase.

Secondly, even though ascorbic acid is rated as one of the least toxic materials, man has been exposed to such low levels of it for so long that suddenly taking comparatively large amounts, orally, may provoke side reactions in a small percentage of certain hypersensitive individuals. Ascorbic acid in the mammals is normally produced in the liver and then poured directly into the bloodstream. This completely avoids the digestive tract, which is normally the route for man. Evidence for these side reactions may be the appearance of gastric distress, vomiting, diarrhea, headache, or skin rashes, all of which disappear on reducing or eliminating the ascorbic acid. Tests should be conducted on these hypersensitive individuals to determine whether their symptoms can be avoided or controlled by substituting the non-acidic sodium ascorbate, by taking the doses with meals, or by gradually building up to the required dosage instead of initially prescribing and starting with the full dosage. In many cases, an initial intolerance to ascorbic acid disappears.

Thirdly, research should also be instituted to determine the validity of the criticism of stone formation as a consequence of high ascorbic acid intakes. This criticism has been leveled in spite of the fact that these high levels have been normal for the mammals for millions of years and the fact that stone formation has been attributed to a *lack* of ascorbic acid (see also Chapter 22). The effect of increased diuresis, due to megascorbic levels, should also be investigated in relation to the mineral metabolism of sodium, potassium, calcium, and magnesium to determine whether increased levels of intake of these essential minerals are required and whether this regimen improves the body's tolerance to sodium.

It is hoped that the research pathways and protocols outlined in the following chapters will serve as a guide for future clinical research to exploit the full therapeutic potential of ascorbic acid for the benefit of man. It is certainly not the intent or the desire of the author that the details of these research proposals be used as the basis for furthering self-medication in any form.

12

THE COMMON COLD

With this chapter, we begin the discussions of the use of ascorbic acid in the treatment of various diseases other than scurvy. We start with the common cold because it is a most annoying ailment and it is one to which everyone is repeatedly exposed. It is also the one with which the author has had the most personal experience. From this personal experience, it is the author's belief that this disease could be eradicated through the proper use of ascorbic acid. It is the purpose of this chapter to tell how this can be done.

Let us first go over some statistics and current research on the common cold and then take a quick look at the medical literature to see what has been done with ascorbic acid in the treatment of the common cold over the last thirty years.

It has been estimated that Americans get about 500 million colds per year. Besides causing acute physical discomfort and taxing the individual's health and stamina, the common cold is the greatest single cause of industrial absenteeism. Its cost to industry appears to be well over five billion dollars a year in lost time and production.

Much research money is being expended now in the hope of developing a vaccine for colds. The probability of developing a useful vaccine is remote because of the large number of different viruses and associated bacteria found in common cold victims. For instance, the rhinoviruses which can be isolated from more than half the adults with common colds comprise about seventy to eighty different serotypes. Since a vaccine is highly specific and only effective against a particular viral strain or bacterial species, it is doubtful whether a polyvalent vaccine would be useful because of this great number of serotypes and the short duration of induced immunity. What is needed, instead, is a wide-spectrum, nontoxic, virucidal, and bactericidal agent. Ascorbic acid fills this bill.

One of the difficulties in common cold research is the general lack of laboratory animals that are susceptible to this disease. Man and apes are reputed to be the only susceptible hosts to this disease. Easily managed laboratory animals such as rats, mice, rabbits, cats, and dogs are said not to catch the disease, thus making laboratory studies very difficult. It is significant that the two species that can catch colds, man and apes, are the two that cannot make their own ascorbic acid.

Shortly after the discovery of ascorbic acid, it was found that it had powerful antiviral activity. This activity was found to be nonspecific and a wide spectrum of viruses were attacked and inactivated. These included the viruses of poliomyelitis, vaccinia, herpes, rabies, foot-and-mouth disease, and tobacco mosaic. The ability of ascorbic acid to inactivate viruses extends to many more and probably covers all the viruses, but these were the ones investigated at this early date. Other workers in the 1930s found that ascorbic acid was capable of inactivating a number of bacterial toxins such as those of diphtheria, tetanus, dysentery, staphylococcus, and anaerobic toxins. These results appeared so promising that, in 1939, they led one worker (1) to state: "Vitamin C, therefore, may truthfully be designated as the 'antitoxic and antiviral' vitamin." And in addition it is relatively harmless to humans.

The medical literature on ascorbic acid and the common cold from 1938 to 1961 can be divided into two groups: one group contains the clinical tests where the ascorbic acid was administered for the treatment of the common cold at dosage rates measured in milligrams per day (one gram or less); the other group contains those where it was given at higher daily dosages. The milligram group found ascorbic acid to be ineffective in the treatment of colds; the higher-dosage group reported more successful results.

Let us skim through this record, covering over a quarter-century, and see what it shows. We will take the inadequate, low-dosage tests first: Berquist (2), in 1940, used 90 milligrams of ascorbic acid per day. Kuttner (3) used 100 milligrams daily on 108 rheumatic children and found no lessening of the incidence of upper-respiratory infections. Cowan, Diehl, and Baker (4) used 200 milligrams per day. Glazebrook and Thomson (5), in 1942, used between 50 and 300 milligrams daily on boys in a large institution. They reported no difference in the incidence of colds and tonsillitis, and the duration of the colds was the same in the group getting the ascorbic acid and that not getting it. The duration of the tonsillitis was longer, however, in the control group, and cases of rheumatic fever and pneumonia developed; but none occurred in the group getting the ascorbic acid. Even at these threshold levels there seemed to be some protection. In 1944 Dahlberg, Engel, and Rydin (6) used 200 milligrams per day on a regiment of Swedish soldiers and reported, "No difference could be found as regards frequency or duration of colds, degrees of fever, etc." Franz and Heyl (7) and Tebrock, Arminio, and Johnston (8), in 1956, both used about 200 milligrams daily in combination with "bioflavanoids," without reporting notable success. At this late date these workers were still proving the pharmacologic fact that you cannot squeeze consistent good therapeutic results from ineffective threshold dosages. Shekhtman (9), in 1961, used 100 milligrams of ascorbic acid for seven months of the year and then 50 milligrams for the rest of the year. He reported a decreased incidence of colds, but the difference was not striking. These are some of the reports of those who used the threshold or "vitamin-like" dosages of milligrams per day. Now, let us turn to the other side of the picture—the group that used higher dosages.

This group includes Ruskin (10) who, in 1938, injected 450 milligrams of calcium ascorbate as soon after the onset of cold symptoms as possible. (This report is included among the higher level group because giving ascorbate by injection is several times more effective than the equivalent dosage by mouth.) In over 2,000 injections there were no complications incident to the injections. Forty-two percent of his patients were completely relieved, usually after the first or second injection. Forty-eight percent were reported as "markedly improved." Ruskin, in his summary, states, "Calcium ascorbate would appear to be practically an abortive in the treatment of the common cold." This statement appeared in 1938, and an astronomical number of colds could have been prevented in the intervening years if only this early work had been followed up. Van Alyea (11), in 1942, found 1 gram a day of ascorbic acid a valuable aid in treating rhinosinusitis. Markwell (12), by 1947, using 3/4 gram or more every three or four hours stated:

My experience seems to show that if the dose is given both early enough and in large enough quantity, the chances of stopping a cold are about fifty-fifty, or perhaps better. It is an amazing and comforting experience to realize suddenly in the middle of the afternoon that no cold is present, after having in the morning expected several days of throat torture. . . .I have never seen any ill effects whatsoever from vitamin C and I do not think there are any. . . .The number of patients who have taken large doses of vitamin C to abort colds during the last three years is considerable—large enough to allow an opinion to be formed, at any rate, as a preliminary to more scientific research.

Albanese (13), in 1947, injected 2 grams of ascorbic acid a day to fight off "la grippe" and reported an immediate alleviation of symptoms, a rapid drop in fever, and shortening of duration of illness. The injections were well tolerated and there were no complications. Albanese reported his observations in the hope that it would stimulate others to try his treatment and obtain additional clinical data. Woolstone (14), in 1954, obtained good results in treating the common cold with 0.8 grams of ascorbic acid hourly and vitamin B complex three times a day. He stated, "Although I can only offer my own observations as proof, the results have been so dramatic that I feel others should be given a chance to try it." Miegl (15), three years later, described the excellent relief of 111 of 132 common cold sufferers in half a day by taking 1 gram of ascorbic acid in tea, three times a day. In 1958 (15), he published another paper extending his previous good results and recommended 2 to 5 grams of ascorbic acid a day for the prophylaxis of respiratory diseases, nosebleeds, radiation sickness, postoperative bleeding, and other conditions. Bessel-Lorch (16) in tests on Berlin high school students at a ski camp gave 1 gram a day to twenty-six students and none to twenty others. After nine days, nine members of the "no-ascorbic" group had fallen ill and only one member of the "ascorbic" group. All students catching colds were given 2 grams of ascorbic acid daily, which produced a general improvement within twenty-four hours so that increased physical exertion could be tolerated without special difficulties. The significant observation was made that, "All participants showed considerable increase in physical stamina under the influence of vitamin C medication." Ritzel (17), in 1961, reported on a larger experiment in a ski camp. One gram of ascorbic acid was given to 139 subjects and 140 others did not receive it. Symptoms were reported in 119 cases from the "no-ascorbic" subjects and 42 cases from the "ascorbic" group. Ritzel stated in his summary, "Statistical evaluation of the results confirmed the efficacy of vitamin C in the prophylaxis and treatment of colds."

There are two things that should be noted in these provocative reports. First, the unheeded appeals for additional extensive clinical research on the high-dosage ascorbic acid treatment of the common cold. Second, the levels of ascorbic acid dosages which were considered "high" by these various authors, who still thought of it as vitamin C, were still far below the dosages that would be considered adequate under the teachings of the genetic disease concept.

In keeping with this new concept, the following regimen for the control of the common cold has been devised and should be subjected to thorough clinical testing. The rationale is based on the known virucidal action of ascorbic acid and the general mammalian response to biochemical stresses. The strategy is to raise the blood and tissue levels of ascorbic acid, by repeated frequent doses, to a point where the virus can no longer survive. It is really difficult to understand how this simple and logical idea has escaped so many investigators for so long. This regime is not untried: the author has been his own "guinea pig" and has not had a cold for nearly two decades. Many of the author's family, colleagues, and friends have volunteered to follow it and have reported successful results. When used as directed it has been practically 100 percent effective.

An individual continuously on the "full correction" regimen of 3 to 5 grams of ascorbic acid daily for an unstressed adult will have a high resistance to infectious respiratory diseases. Should the exposure to the infectious agent be unduly heavy or some other uncorrected biochemical stresses be imposed, the infecting virus may gain a foothold and start developing. Treatment is instituted at the very first indication of the cold starting, because it is much easier to abort an incipient cold than to try to treat an advanced case. If a known heavy exposure to the infectious agent is experienced, such as close contacts with a coughing and sneezing cold sufferer, then extra prophylactic doses of several grams of ascorbic acid, several times a day, may be taken without waiting for cold symptoms to develop.

At the first symptoms of a developing cold I take about 1.5 to 2.0 grams of ascorbic acid, dissolved in a couple of ounces of water, unsweetened or sweetened to taste. Within twenty minutes to half an hour another dose is ingested and this is repeated at twenty-minute to half-hour intervals. Usually by the third dose the virus has been effectively inactivated, and usually no further cold symptoms will appear. I watch for any delayed symptoms and, if any become evident, I take further doses. If the start of this regimen is delayed and it is instituted only after the virus has spread throughout the body, the results may not be so dramatic, but ascorbic acid will nevertheless be of great benefit. Continued dosages at one- or two-hour intervals will shorten the duration of the attack, often to a day. The great advantage of this common cold therapy is that it utilizes a normal body constituent rather than some foreign toxic material. This regime should be the subject of large-scale, long-range clinical studies in order to establish its efficacy and safety, and to provide the data required by medicine for any new suggested therapy.

In 1966, this regime was sent to Dr. Linus Pauling. As a result of his successful personal experience and other work, he published, in 1970, the book (18) *Vitamin C and the Common Cold.* This volume, the first published book in the new fields of megascorbic prophylaxis and megascorbic therapy, gives a more detailed and practical account of the use of ascorbic acid for this condition than is possible in the space of this short chapter.

With the publication of this book, there was a rash of unjustified criticism heaped upon Dr. Pauling by the medical establishment as well as the lay press. In the second edition of this book, published by Bantam Books in 1971, Dr. Pauling answers these criticisms. Chapter 12 ends with the statement:

> With the increasing recognition of the value of vitamin C and the increasing use of this natural and essential substance to strengthen the body's defenses against infections, this universal scourge, the common cold, can be brought under control.

Up to the date of the publication of this book, the author is not aware of any clinical tests planned or started that follow the suggested regimen of: 1. long-term correction of hypoascorbemia to improve resistance against the cold virus, and 2. massive virucidal therapy with ascorbic acid once the symptoms of the cold appear.

13

VIRAL INFECTION

The many different contagious diseases that afflict man may be divided and classified according to the nature and characteristics of the infecting agent that causes the disease. Three groups are generally recognized: the viral diseases, the bacterial infections, and the diseases caused by more advanced types of parasitic agents.

It so happens that this classification also denotes the relative size and complexity of the infectious agents. The viruses are the simplest and most primitive forms; in fact, they are sort of transitional substances between living and nonliving matter. They cause a wide variety of diseases such as poliomyelitis, measles, smallpox, chicken pox, influenza, "shingles," mumps, and rabies. The common cold, discussed in the previous chapter, is a virus disease, although various bacteria generally infect the weakened tissues as secondary invaders.

When a virus infects a mammal and gains a foothold in the mammalian body, the mammal reacts by showing the symptoms of the disease and at the same time organizes its own biochemical defenses against the virus. In nearly all mammals, this biochemical defensive reaction is at least twofold: the victim starts to produce antibodies against the virus and also increases the rate of ascorbic acid synthesis in its liver. This is the normal mammalian reaction to the disease process, except in those species, like man, that cannot manufacture their own ascorbic acid.

Let us see what a review of the medical literature reveals about megascorbic therapy and viral disease:

Poliomyelitis

The application of ascorbic acid in the treatment of poliomyelitis is an incredible story of high hopes that end in disappointment, of blunders and lack of insight, of misguided labors and erroneous hypothesis. And then, when a worker finally seemed to be on the right path and had demonstrated success, hardly anyone believed his results, which were systematically ignored.

Within two years after the discovery of ascorbic acid, Jungeblut (1) showed that ascorbic acid would inactivate the virus of poliomyelitis. This was followed, in 1936-1937, in rapid succession by other workers showing similar inactivation of other viruses: by Holden et al. (2), using the herpes virus; by Kligler and Bernkopf (3), on the vaccinia virus, by Langenbusch and Enderling (4), with the virus of hoof-and-mouth disease; by Amato (5), on the rabies virus; by Lominski (6), using bacteriophage; and by Lojkin and Martin (7), with the tobacco mosaic disease virus. Thus, at this early date it was established that ascorbic acid had the potential of being a wide-spectrum antiviral agent. Here was a new "magic bullet" that was effective against a wide variety of viruses and was known to be completely harmless. Materials with such exciting properties do not happen often and a tremendous amount of research time should have been expended in tracking it down in minute detail, but let us see what happened.

The reader should realize that this work was being carried out in the pre-Salk days. Then, all a doctor could do in a polio case was apply symptomatic relief and hope for the best. An epidemic could run its course without much interference from medicine and an effective, harmless virucide would have been a priceless commodity. Jungeblut (8) continued his work and published a series of papers from 1936 to 1939 in which he showed that the administra-

tion of ascorbic acid to monkeys infected with poliomyelitis produced a distinct reduction in the severity of the disease and enhanced their resistance to it. Sabin (9), attempting to reproduce
Jungeblut's work on monkeys, failed to obtain these partially successful results. In further efforts to explain their variable clinical
results, both scientists got bogged down chasing the technical details
of the tests. It may be easy for us to look back now and say that
the size and the frequency of the dosages were insufficient to
maintain high levels of ascorbic acid in the blood during the
incubation of the disease. The upshot was that the negative findings
of Sabin effectively stifled further research in this field for a decade.

In 1949, the first of a remarkable series of papers appeared.
Klenner (10) described his successful treatment of poliomyelitis,
as well as a variety of many other viral infections, using ascorbic
acid. He gave the rationale for his treatment, his technique in
detail, and his dramatic case histories. Klenner realized that the
secret was in the massive doses he employed, and he tried to impart
this knowledge to an unbelieving profession. In his 1952 paper,
Klenner further discussed his ascorbic acid treatment of polio and
comments on Jungeblut's earlier work, stating:

> His results were indecisive because the amount of vitamin C
> given was inadequate to cope with the degree of infection.
> Sabin's results were not as suggestive as Jungeblut's because he,
> Sabin, used a greater dose of virus and less vitamin C.

Klenner's suggested optimal dosage rate for virus infections,
calculated on the basis of a 70-kilogram (154-pound) adult, was
4.5 to 17.5 grams of ascorbic acid given every two to four hours
around the clock (27 to 210 grams per day). This amount goes far
beyond anything that had been previously tried. He records one
successful case history after another in these papers, as well as in
his 1953 report. His results indeed proved that ascorbic acid was a
harmless and effective wide-spectrum virucidal agent. If high blood
and tissue levels of ascorbic acid are continuously maintained, an
extremely unfavorable environment for viral growth and reproduction is created in the human body.

Two other papers appeared in 1952, in which ascorbic acid was
used in the therapy of poliomyelitis at daily doses below those
recommended by Klenner. Gsell and Kalt (11), using 5 to 25

grams per day, reported that there were no definite effects on the course of the disease. Besides using lower dosages, they also started this treatment on the majority of their patients only after they had had the disease for at least four days. Baur (12), using 10 to 20 grams per day, was able to report beneficial results in shortening the fever and convalescent time.

Greer (13), in 1955, using doses in Klenner's recommended range (50 to 80 grams per day), recorded the good clinical results he had obtained in five serious cases of poliomyelitis.

Over the years, the emphasis of medical research on poliomyelitis has shifted toward the development of vaccines. These are now widely used and have the disease under control. But a polio vaccine is only effective against the polio virus and has no action on the viruses of other diseases. The main value of Klenner's work is in showing that any active viral disease can be successfully brought under control with ascorbic acid if the proper large doses are used. It is inconceivable, but true, that Klenner's pioneering work has been almost completely ignored; no large-scale tests have been made to explore the exciting possibilities of his provocative clinical results. Millions of dollars of research money have been spent in unsuccessful attempts to find a nontoxic, effective virucide and all sorts of exotic chemicals have been tried. All the while, harmless, inexpensive, and nontoxic ascorbic acid has been within easy reach of these investigators. It might prove to be the "magic bullet" for the control of the viral diseases.

Hepatitis

Soon after the discovery of ascorbic acid, Bessey and coworkers (14), in 1933, showed that guinea pigs deprived of ascorbic acid developed a fatty degeneration of the liver. Ten years later, Russell and Calloway (15) also showed pathologic changes in the livers of guinea pigs with scurvy. Willis (16), in 1957, further investigated and extended these earlier observations and demonstrated the vital importance of ascorbic acid in maintaining healthy liver tissue free of cirrhotic, degenerative changes.

Ascorbic acid should, therefore, be twice as sound for use in the treatment of the viral liver disease, viral hepatitis. When used at the necessary high dosages it should inactivate the hepatitis virus and it should also act on the liver tissue to prevent degenerative changes. In 1954, Bauer and Staub (17) observed good results in the treatment of viral hepatitis with the use of 10 grams of ascorbic acid per day. It accelerated the disappearance of the symptoms of the disease and shortened the duration of the illness. Earlier, in 1937, Spengler (18), using only 100 milligrams per day by injection in a case of liver cirrhosis brought on by the toxemia of pregnancy, noted ascorbic acid's diuretic effect, which helped clear up the disease, and reported good recovery. Twenty years later in Germany, Kirchmair (19) used 10 grams of ascorbic acid daily for five days on sixty-three children with hepatitis and found marked improvement, weight gain and good appetite in the first few days, rapid disappearance of jaundice and half the hospitalization time. The swelling of the liver, which normally took 30 days to subside, only took nine days with ascorbic acid. In 1960, Calleja and Brooks (20) reported successful treatment with 5 grams of ascorbic acid a day for twenty-four days in a refractory case of hepatitis that did not respond to other medication. Baetgen (21), giving 10 grams of ascorbic acid a day to 245 children with hepatitis, obtained results similar to Kirchmair's, with rapid recovery and better tissue repair. Dalton (22), in 1962, also reported dramatic and rapid recovery of a case of hepatitis.

In these clinical reports on hepatitis, the doses of ascorbic acid were below the range postulated by Klenner and also below the quantity considered necessary by the genetic disease concepts. The provocative clinical results reported in the medical literature have not been extended or explored. Further intensive clinical research is needed on the use of ascorbic acid at the proper high-dosage rate for the control of this serious liver disease and also for the prevention and therapy of the degenerative, cirrhotic liver changes that occur, for instance, from the excessive use of alcohol. It is tragic that organizations concerned with alcoholism have not picked up these exciting leads for further exploration to prevent the degenerative liver changes which cause such misery and death to so many. The long-term preventive use of only 10 grams of ascorbic acid a day may be sufficient.

Herpes

This is an acute inflammatory affliction of the skin or mucous membrane and is known in many different forms, all annoying and some quite serious. Two common forms are "fever blisters," or herpes simplex, a more or less serious condition depending upon the location of the "blisters," while "shingles," or herpes zoster, is a serious and painful disorder which seems to follow and inflame the paths of certain nerves. The virus appears to reside in the skin and the disease starts when the victim is exposed to excessive stresses such as overexposure to sunlight or poisons, infections, or physical or emotional stresses. These are all conditions where ascorbic acid is at a low ebb in the body and this may be part of the triggering mechanism that starts the disease.

It was shown early by Holden & Molloy (2) that ascorbic acid inactivated the herpes virus. Clinical tests conducted later indicated provocative improvements. Dainow (23), in 1943, reported successful treatment of 14 cases of "shingles" with injections of ascorbic acid; Zureick (24), in 1950, treated 327 cases of "shingles" and claimed cures in all in 3 days of injections of ascorbic acid; Klenner (10), in 1949, injected eight "shingle" patients with ascorbic acid and seven claimed cessation of pain within two hours after the first injection. Seven also showed drying of the blisters within one day and in three days were clear of the lesions.

Again, no large-scale testings have been made to verify these exciting results, with the numerically and statistically significant volume of cases that medicine demands before it accepts a treatment. This is another job for a government-supported program, but no one has picked it up and carried it through.

Other Viral Diseases

Klenner (25), in 1948, and Dalton (22), in 1962, reported their successful experiences with *virus pneumonia* treated with ascorbic acid in 42 cases and 3 cases, respectively. Paez de la Torre (26), in 1945, found good results in *measles* in children. Klenner (10), in 1949, successfully used ascorbic acid as a prophylactic in a measles epidemic and gave a dramatic case history in his 1953 paper in the treatment of a ten-month-old baby with measles. Zureick (24), in 1950, treated seventy-one cases of *chicken pox* with ascorbic acid and Klenner (10), in 1949, also mentions the good response he obtained in this disease.

Klenner also cites the dramatic results he obtained in *virus encephalitis* and also in 33 cases of *mumps* and many cases of *influenza.* Vargas Magne (27), in 1963, treated 130 cases of influenza for one to three days using up to 45 grams of ascorbic acid. The patients were both male and female, aged ten to forty years; 114 recovered and 16 did not respond. The present direction of the research on influenza in this country is oriented to lead to the development of a vaccine. There appears to be no provision in this research program for testing massive doses of ascorbic acid in the prevention or treatment of influenza.

Amato (5), in 1937, found that the *rabies* virus could be inactivated with ascorbic acid. A search of the literature revealed no further work in the thirty-five years since this paper originally appeared. Here could be the nucleus of a possible harmless treatment of this fatal disease if the necessary work would be conducted using large, continuing doses of ascorbic acid. There is a very great need for a relatively harmless treatment of rabies as the present therapy is almost as bad as the disease. This is certainly an area where more work should be done, and done soon in view of the recent findings of large reservoirs of the rabies virus in bats (28, 29).

Still another area, long unexplored, is in the prophylaxis and treatment of *smallpox.* A 1937 report by Kligler and Bernkopf (3) stated that ascorbic acid inactivates the vaccinia virus. Nothing further can be found in the medical literature to indicate the use of ascorbic acid in the related disease, smallpox.

Infectious mononucleosis, usually a long drawn-out disease, should be amenable to treatment with ascorbic acid, and one case, with dramatic recovery, has been reported (22).

Many of the papers cited above end with the plea for further work on a larger scale to evaluate thoroughly the use of massive doses of ascorbic acid in the therapy of the viral diseases. These pleas have gone unheeded. Was it because there was no rationale for the high dosage rates under the old vitamin C theory? The new genetic disease concept now supplies a logical rationale for the use of these high doses of ascorbic acid in therapy. From the work already conducted, it would appear that ascorbic acid is a most valuable weapon in the fight against the viral diseases when used under the proper conditions. How valuable it is we shall never know unless large-scale clinical tests are undertaken by our presently constituted public health agencies and publicly supported health foundations. Let us see if the record of the next decade is better than the last.

14

BACTERIAL INFECTION

In this chapter we will discuss the use of ascorbic acid in the treatment of the infectious diseases caused by pathogenic bacteria. These include tuberculosis, pneumonia, pertussis (whooping cough), leprosy, typhoid fever, dysentery, and other infections.

There is a tremendous volume of medical literature relating to the treatment of infectious bacterial diseases with ascorbic acid. Much of it appeared in the early days, not too long after the discovery of ascorbic acid, because these early workers had high hopes for the therapeutic potency of ascorbic acid in a wide variety of diseases. Before discussing these clinical tests we will review some elementary facts of pharmacology that seem to have escaped nearly all of these investigators for the past thirty years.

A substance that has the property of killing bacteria is called a "germicide" or "bactericide." The germicidal potency will vary from substance to substance. Because of this variation, a certain specific minimum concentration must be maintained, under stated conditions, for the substance to exert its killing or bactericidal powers. If this minimum concentration is lowered somewhat, so that the killing power is lost, the substance may still be able to have a growth-inhibiting, or bacteriostatic, effect. At these lower levels, the substance prevents the bacteria from growing without actually killing them. Reducing the concentration of a bacteriostatic substance further could permit the bacteria to start growing. Thus, we have certain levels of concentration where the bacteria can be killed, their growth inhibited, or just not affected at all. These simple facts have been known since the nineteenth century.

It has also been known for some time that ascorbic acid has bacteriostatic and bactericidal properties. It was shown (1), in 1941, that various microorganisms could be inhibited by ascorbic acid at 2 milligram percent (mg %)—that is, 2 parts of ascorbic acid in 100,000 parts of bacterial suspension. The bacteria included *Staphylococcus aureus* (the pus organism), *B. typhosus* (the germ causing typhoid fever), *B. coli* (the organism from sewage), and *B. subtilis* (a nonpathogenic bacteria). At 5 mg % *B. diphtheriae* was inhibited as well as *Streptococcus hemolyticus* (the cause of many serious infections). Several authors worked with the tuberculosis organism, which was found to be particularly susceptible to attack by ascorbic acid. Boissevain and Spillane (2), in 1937, found a bacteriostatic effect at 1 mg %; Sirsi (3), in 1952, reported 10 mg % to be bactericidal against virulent strains of *M. tuberculosis* and bacteriostatic at 1 mg %; Myrvik et al. (4), in 1954, also showed the bacteriostatic action of ascorbic acid and confirmed earlier observations that the urine from subjects taking ascorbic acid acquired the property of inhibiting the growth of the tubercle bacilli.

Using these figures, we can make a rough calculation of how much ascorbic acid would be needed to reach a bacteriostatic or a bactericidal level in the body. If we take 10 mg % as our desired level and assume that the ascorbic acid would be equally distributed throughout the whole body and the patient's weight is 70 kilograms (154 pounds), then the *minimum* initial dose required would be 7 grams, or 7,000 milligrams. Actually, much more would be required each day, for a number of reasons, in order to maintain a 10 mg % concentration; but this figure is good enough for our comparison with the actual amounts used in the clinical tests. It is apparent that none of the investigators paused to make this calculation before planning their tests because the dosages they used are of a completely different order of magnitude—so low as to be obviously inadequate.

Let us now look into some other useful properties of ascorbic acid. Certain bacteria, during their growth, elaborate and secrete deadly poisons or toxins. In some of the infectious diseases, the most distressing symptoms and toxic effects, such as the choking of diphtheria or the muscle spasms of tetanus, or lockjaw, are caused by these toxins. The toxin produced by bacteria causing a type of food poisoning, the botulinus toxin, is one of the most powerful and deadly poisons known to man. The lethal dose is so small it is invisible to the naked eye.

It was early found that ascorbic acid had the power to neutralize, inactivate, and render harmless a wide variety of these bacterial toxins: diphtheria (5) (Harde and Phillippe, 1934; Jungeblut and Zwemer, 1935; Sigal and King, 1937; Kligler et al., 1937); tetanus (6) (Jungeblut, 1937; Kligler et al., 1938; Schulze and Hecht, 1937; Kuribayashi et al., 1963; Dey, 1966); staphylococcus (7) (Kodama and Kojima, 1939); dysentery (8) (Takahashi, 1938). In 1934, the unusual resistance of the mouse to diphtheria infections was attributed to its ability to synthesize rapidly its own ascorbic acid, while the guinea pig's ready susceptibility to this disease (like man's) was attributed to its inability to replenish its store of ascorbic acid.

Another of the body's defenses against invading pathogenic bacteria is the mobilization of the white blood cells in the site of the infection. These white blood cells actually physically attack the bacteria, engulf them, and digest and destroy them. This process of actually eating the bacteria is called "phagocytosis." The white blood cells are really the scavengers and garbage men of the tissues. This important bodily defense is an ascorbic acid-dependent process. The phagocytic activity depends on the amount of ascorbic acid in the blood and tissues. If the ascorbic acid levels are too low the white blood cells will not attack the invading bacteria, nor ingest or digest them. The fact that phagocytosis proceeds poorly or not at all is a major reason for the increased susceptibility to infections in the prescorbutic or scorbutic state.

Cottingham and Mills (8), in 1943, showed this necessity for the presence of ascorbic acid in maintaining phagocytotic activity of the white blood cells. In their tests there was a marked reduction in this vital defensive measure with ascorbic acid deficiency. This important discovery made no impression at the time. Nearly three decades later this effect was "rediscovered" by DeChatelet et al. (8) and received wide newspaper coverage.

To summarize—in ascorbic acid we have a theoretically ideal weapon in the fight against the infectious diseases:

1. It is bacteriostatic or bactericidal and will prevent the growth or kill the pathogenic organisms.
2. It detoxicates and renders harmless the bacterial toxins and poisons.
3. It controls and maintains phagocytosis.
4. It is harmless and nontoxic and can be administered in the large doses needed to accomplish the above effects without danger to the patient.

A great volume of work with the infectious diseases was initiated soon after the discovery of ascorbic acid, because of the long-standing suspicion of a causal connection between scurvy and infections. Scurvy and the prescorbutic state were known to lower the body's resistance and predispose both humans and guinea pigs to the infectious diseases (9) (Faulkner and Taylor, 1937; Harris et al., 1937; Perla and Marmorsten, 1937). This was in the days before the antibiotics and sulfonamides, when medicine's armament against infections was still rather primitive and nonspecific and the infections took a high toll in suffering and death. The early workers were intrigued with this newly discovered substance and its unique therapeutic powers, and thought it would be a mighty weapon in the fight against infectious diseases. Hundreds of papers were published; the few cited below are merely a sampling.

Tuberculosis

The medical literature of the two decades before the discovery of ascorbic acid contains many pertinent empirical observations and animal experiments on the relationship among scurvy, tuberculosis, and vitamin C. As early as 1933, McConkey and Smith (10) fed guinea pigs tuberculous sputum daily. One group of animals was maintained on a diet partially deficient in ascorbic acid and in the other group each animal received 2 teaspoons of tomato juice daily as their source of ascorbic acid (about 2 milligrams a day). McConkey got the idea for this test from his earlier observation of the permanent improvement of hospitalized patients with intestinal tuberculosis on being given tomato juice in addition to their regular hospital fare. Of the thirty-seven animals on the partially deficient diet, 26 developed ulcerative intestinal tuberculosis, while only two of the thirty-five tomato juice animals succumbed, despite the extremely low levels of ascorbic acid used. Other workers (11) confirmed these results (de Savitsch et al., 1934) using 2 teaspoons of orange juice per animal per day, and Greene et al., in 1936, published confirmatory data. Birkhaug, in 1938, in a very complete series of tests on guinea pigs, using only 10 milligrams of ascorbic acid a day for a 300-gram guinea pig (equivalent to 2300 milligrams for a human adult), came to the following conclusions:

Our study has shown that by compensating for the inevitable state of hypovitaminosis C which occurs in progressive tuberculosis, we render the animal organism more resistant against the inflammatory-necrotizing effect of tuberculosis and the initial invasive onslaught of virulent tubercle bacilli.

As reported in two short papers, in 1936 and 1939, Heise et al. (12), using 20 milligrams of ascorbic acid a day subcutaneously, found no influence on the course of the infection. However, when the experimental conditions are examined, it is found that while they had given twice as much ascorbic acid as Birkhaug had, they had also increased their inoculation of highly virulent tuberculosis bacteria to *20* to *600* times more than Birkhaug had used. It is quite evident why they did not confirm Birkhaug's work: they expected too much from too little ascorbic acid.

Good results with ascorbic acid in protecting guinea pigs against the effects of tuberculosis were also reported by workers (13) in Germany, the United States, Denmark, and other countries.

Many papers appeared which showed the increased need for ascorbic acid under the heavy biochemical stresses of the tuberculosis infection (14). In a five-year follow-up study of 1,100 men originally free of pulmonary tuberculosis, 28 cases of tuberculosis developed; all the cases came from the group whose ascorbic acid blood levels were substandard (15).

Clinical tests reported from 1935 to 1939 include the following (16): Hasselbach, using 100 milligrams of ascorbic acid a day for treatment, reported some favorable effects. Radford and coworkers gave 500 milligrams a day in cases of advanced and fibroid tuberculosis and obtained improvement in the blood picture. Borsalino, who injected 100 milligrams a day, controlled hemorrhaging and improved the general condition of his patients. Martin and Heise, using 200 milligrams a day, did not obtain any evidence of a beneficial effect. Petter administered 150 milligrams of ascorbic acid a day to forty-nine tuberculous adults, of which thirty improved, twelve showed no change, and seven were definitely worse; of twenty-four tuberculous children, twenty-one improved, one showed no change, and two were worse. The higher percentage of improved patients among the children was, no doubt, due to their higher dosage per unit of body weight. Albrecht injected 100 milligrams a day and obtained improvement in appetite, well-being, weight gain, blood picture, and temperature. Josewich gave 100 to 150 milligrams a day and reported practically no effect on his tuberculous patients. Baksh and Rabbani injected 500 milligrams a day for 4 days and gave 150 to 200 milligrams orally for the next 6 weeks. They reported it was a valuable adjuvant in treatment.

In spite of this lack of any notable or outstanding success and of the marginal (at best) responses they were obtaining with these low doses, the tests continued at the same low levels. The dogma of the vitamin theory kept these clinicians from thinking of ascorbic acid as an antibiotic and using it at the necessary antibiotic dosages. A sampling of this continuing useless work appearing in the 1940s follows (17): Erwin et al., and Kaplan et al., administered 100 to 200 milligrams a day and both reported no significant favorable effects in tuberculosis. Sweaney et al., giving about 200 milligrams a day in 3 series of patients could report no outstanding success. Vitorero and Doyle injected 500 to 600 milligrams of ascorbic acid a day initially, which was reduced to 400 milligrams as improvement was shown, and then further reduced to 200 milligrams a day. They were quite positive about the benefits of this medication in their few cases and recommended its use in intestinal tuberculosis. Bogen et al., treating 200 patients divided into several groups in a sanatorium with 150 milligrams of ascorbic acid a day, reported subjective improvement in the patients and visible improvement in the tuberculous lesions. They stated that vitamin C was by no means a cure for tuberculosis, but they recommended its "abundant administration," which to them meant 150 milligrams a day. They attached no importance to ascorbic acid's controlling of the symptoms of tuberculosis, but said that many patients expressed a feeling of increased well-being. Rudra and Roy, in 1946, and Babbar, in 1948, found the same borderline type of improvements using 250 milligrams and 200 miliigrams of ascorbic acid per day, respectively.

There were many more reports in this sickening mass of continued repetition of ineffectual clinical tests where the investigators were correcting a nutritional deficiency instead of using ascorbic acid to actually combat the disease. At last, in 1948, Charpy (18) got the idea that the doses previously used were too low and conducted a test using 15 grams (15,000 milligrams) of ascorbic acid a day on six tuberculous patients. But even this test was bungled: the six patients selected for the test were terminal tuberculosis cases expected to die shortly and, in fact, one of the patients did die before the test could really get under way. Of the other five, they were still alive six to eight months later, had gained from twenty to seventy pounds in weight, were no longer bedridden, and had had a spectacular transformation of their general condition. Charpy stated that while there was not much modification in the physical appearance of their tuberculous lesions, "they gave the impression of becoming in some way unaware of the enormous tuberculous lesions they harbored." He noted that each patient had taken about 3 kilograms (3,000,000 milligrams) of ascorbic acid during the test with safety and perfect tolerance. He also indicated that further work was being done, but a search of the subsequent medical literature failed to reveal any further reports by Charpy or by anyone else using these large doses. No one has taken these exciting results and further explored their possibilities.

The record of the clinical work conducted on the use of ascorbic acid in the treatment of tuberculosis is, indeed, incredible. After thirty years, the crucial and meaningful clinical tests at high dosages have still not been conducted. Uncounted lives have been lost; immeasurable suffering endured; and time, energy, and research money wasted in chasing a will-o'-the-wisp by minds looking for a therapeutic effect, but bound by the narrow confines of a vitamin theory. It is unbelievable that so many workers for so long a time could not have suspected the possible reason for their uniform lack of success. To these workers, doses of a few hundred milligrams of ascorbic acid a day were considered "high" because they looked upon it as a *vitamin* and not as an *antibiotic*. The correct employment of ascorbic acid could relegate the White Plague to oblivion.

Pneumonia

Hochwald used injections of 500 milligrams of ascorbic acid every one-and-a-half hours in croupous pneumonia until the fever subsided. He noted a quicker disappearance of fever and local symptoms and a normalization of blood counts; the disease could practically be cut short the first day. Gander and Niederberger, injecting 500 milligrams intramuscularly and then 900 milligrams orally in the next 3 hours, reported remarkable improvement during the disease and in convalescence. Gunzel and Kroehnert had good results at 1,000 to 1,600 milligrams a day and some failures at 500 milligrams a day. Kienart, Szirmai, and Stein reported good results in pneumonia as well as Biilmann, who injected 500 milligrams of ascorbic acid every 3 hours. Chacko injected 1 gram every 4 hours into infants with pneumonia with excellent results (19).

The encouraging results in pneumonia were obtained using ascorbic acid at levels, which, though "genetically" low, were still higher than those used in tuberculosis. Most of this work was done in the pre-antibiotic era, when a good treatment for penumonia was vitally needed, and yet ascorbic acid never was widely used or even properly explored for the therapy of pneumonia. Even now, when antibiotics are dominating the field of pneumonia therapy, ascorbic acid in large doses still has a useful function as an adjuvant to antibiotic therapy. In large doses, it will potentiate the effectiveness of the antibiotic and make it possible to use smaller doses of the expensive antibiotic. It will also detoxicate the harmful side reactions incident to the use of these antibiotics, thus assuring the patient a better chance of survival. More work should be conducted in these areas.

Pertussis (Whooping Cough)

In 1936, it was shown that ascorbic acid at 8 mg percent had an inhibiting effect on the growth of the germ causing whooping cough (20). In the same year Otani (20) demonstrated ascorbic acid's ability to neutralize the toxin of the whooping cough bacillus and its usefulness in the management of whooping cough by injection. In a later paper, in 1939, he used 5 to 12 injections of 100 to 200 milligrams of ascorbic acid on 109 cases of whooping cough. He summed up his tests by stating, "the treatment with vitamin C for the whooping cough is a new method superior to all other treatments given heretofore for the patients." He found "remarkable efficiency" in 40 cases (36.7 percent), "some efficiency" in 49 cases (45 percent) and in the remaining 20 cases (18.3 percent) "no efficiency at all." In this latter group, the majority of the patients had other complications, such as tuberculosis, measles, influenza, tonsillitis, etc., and this alone should have indicated to subsequent workers the need for increased and higher dosages. But no, the testing at these inadequate "nutritional" levels of treatment proceeded unabated.

Four papers appeared in 1937–38 (21) from such widely separated places as Canada, Germany, England, and Kansas using doses varying from 100 to 350 milligrams a day and reporting some marginal measure of success. Gairdner, in 1938, using what he believed to be unusually large doses of ascorbic acid (200 milligrams a day for the first week, 150 milligrams a day for the second week, and 100 milligrams a day thereafter), found no differences between the course of the whooping cough in twenty-one vitamin C–treated cases and twenty control cases without the vitamin C. Sessa (22), in 1940, injecting 100 milligrams a day (in some serious cases 250 or 500 milligrams) into infants, found a reduction in convulsive coughing and a quicker recovery and considered it a valuable therapeutic measure.

Another overlooked clue that should have provided these workers with an important lead that their dosages were inadequate was the fact that infants generally responded to the ascorbic acid treatments much better than adults. This was due to the smaller size of the infants so that they actually received a considerably larger dose of ascorbic acid per unit of body weight.

Meier (22), in 1945, found a reduction in coughing and that the coughing spells were more easily tolerated, *especially in infants.* There was general improvement, the children looked better and were more quiet, their appetite increased and vomiting disappeared. He gave 500 milligrams by injection supplemented by six 300-milligram tablets orally, the dosage totaling 2,300 milligrams daily for the first few days. Meier's consistently greater success is probably due to his use of slightly higher dosage levels than his predecessors.

Pfeiffer (23), in 1947, injected 500 milligrams daily, intramuscularly, and also supplemented this with ascorbic acid tablets, orally, but she failed to state how much the tablets contained. She reported no success.

The last paper we will discuss comes from Holland (23), where 500 milligrams of ascorbic acid was used per day either by injection or orally for the first week. Then the dosage was reduced stepwise. In the ninety children treated, the duration of the illness was fifteen days for the injected group, twenty days for the oral group, and thirty-four days for the control group, which received vaccine. He stated, "Ascorbic acid given in the catarrhal stages prevented the convulsive stage in 75 percent of the cases, whereas the number of complications were negligible."

This review shows that the results of the work on whooping cough, covering a period of about fifteen years, provided some variable relief, but resulted mostly in inconclusive and confusing reports. The crucial experiment, where ascorbic acid was used at the necessary antibiotic and antitoxic levels of many grams a day, was never conducted.

Leprosy

Leprosy is a disease of much wider occurrence than is generally supposed. It is not limited to the undeveloped areas of the Far East but is also present on the American continents.

Ascorbic acid has been tried in the treatment of leprosy over a period of many years. Bechelli (Brazil 1939), using 50 to 100 milligrams by intramuscular injection, reported good results in over half of the twenty cases he treated. Gatti and Gaona (Paraguay 1939) noted improvements in two cases of leprosy using daily injections of 100 milligrams of ascorbic acid for several weeks. Ugarriza (Paraguay 1939) obtained relief in leprous septicemia with eight 50-milligram tablets of ascorbic acid orally. Ferreira (Brazil 1950) at the Santa Isabel Leper Colony found that the daily injection of 500 milligrams of ascorbic acid improved the well-being of the lepers, their appetite increased, they gained weight, they had fewer nosebleeds and it improved their tolerance to other antileprosy treatments. He stated that it was a valuable auxiliary medication. Floch and Sureau (France 1952), using daily injections of 500 milligrams over long periods, observed favorable results in the tuberculoid form of the disease. They also reported better results at twice the daily dosage (1 gram a day) and suggested that it would be interesting to continue their work at "2 or even 4 grams daily," but apparently this was never done by them or anyone else (24). From the beneficial results obtained thus far from doses that were obviously too low, the odds would seem to favor success at proper dosage levels. Who will make these tests and when?

Typhoid Fever

By the strict use of control measures, such as improvements in methods of sewage disposal, protection of communal water supplies, pasteurization of selected foods, and exclusion of typhoid carriers from food handling professions, good protection against typhoid fever is obtained. However, sporadic outbreaks do occur in spite of continued alertness: for instance, the 280-case outbreak in Zermatt, Switzerland, in 1963; the 400-case epidemic in Aberdeen, Scotland, in 1964; and the Atlanta, Georgia, episode in the same year involving 15 cases and 1 death. In the United States, typhoid vaccine inoculations are ordinarily given only to members of the armed forces and to persons traveling abroad. The home folks, not in the armed forces, are left unprotected against this serious disease which, even with the newer antibiotic treatments, has a mortality rate of 4.5 percent and a relapse rate of 15 to 20 percent.

In 1937 Farah (25), in England, reported outstanding success in reducing mortality and duration of illness in 18 cases of typhoid fever treated with ascorbic acid and cortin. Szirmai (19), in 1940, used ascorbic acid injections in severe cases of typhoid fever, 300 milligrams a day, which completely prevented the intestinal hemorrhaging. In 1943, in a comprehensive paper, Drummond (25) published the very successful results of his treatment of 106 cases of typhoid fever with 1,200 milligrams of ascorbic acid daily, 400 milligrams by injection and 800 milligrams orally.

The results obtained in these early tests warrant the futher exploration of the use of the necessary high doses of ascorbic acid in the prophylaxis and treatment of this and related diseases, either as the sole medicament or as an adjuvant with other antibiotic therapy. While the incidence of typhoid fever, caused by the bacterium, *Salmonella typhosa,* has been declining in the last twenty years, other related diseases caused by similar species of Salmonella have shown very sharp increases. These are the typhoidlike food-borne infections commonly regarded as "food poisoning." The Salmonella organisms are the type that secrete poisonous toxins which are in part responsible for the virulence of the infection. Ascorbic acid, at the proper high dosages, should be particularly valuable in these Salmonella infections because of its antibiotic effect and its toxin-neutralizing powers.

Dysentery

This is another infectious disease caused by poor sanitation, and the infectious agent is an amoeba. A controlled study has been made of ascorbic acid in guinea pigs experimentally infected with the amoeba of human origin (26). Some of the animals were maintained on an ascorbic acid-deficient diet and others were given 20 milligrams of ascorbic acid every other day (this is a nutritional dosage, not a therapeutic antibiotic level). Higher infectivity, mortality rates, and increased severity of the disease were found in the animals maintained without added ascorbic acid. Two Russian workers (26), in 1957, found a definite relationship between the clinical manifestations of dysentery and the ascorbic acid levels in 106 patients. In the deficient patients there were more hemorrhages and frequent slimy-bloody stools. They only used 150 milligrams a day to try to control the disease. In 1958, another Russian paper appeared in which 500 milligrams a day were used. When the ascorbic acid was combined with other treatments, it rapidly eliminated the clinical symptoms of severe dysentery, led to more favorable progress, and shortened the duration of the illness. The favorable clinical responses at the submarginal levels used in this work would indicate good promise of greater success in any future trial of the megascorbic therapy of this disease.

Other Infections

Typhus is a disease caused by minute microorganisms called "rickettsias" which occupy a position between bacteria and viruses. They are usually transmitted to man by lice, fleas, mites, or ticks. Other rickettsial diseases are *Rocky Mountain spotted fever* or *tick fever* of the eastern and northwestern United States, *trench fever* of central Europe, *tsutsugamushi* of the Asiastic-Pacific area, and *rickettsialpox* of New York City and Boston. If megascorbic therapy is found useful in one of the rickettsial diseases, it will probably control all. Szirmai (19) had been using ascorbic acid in the treatment of typhus since 1936, with serious cases getting 300-milligram injections of ascorbic acid once or twice daily in addition to 100 milligrams orally three times a day. Dujardin (27) noted that a study of typhus had been made in a Casablanca hospital using 8 to 16 grams of ascorbic acid per day. The use of high doses of ascorbic acid in these serious diseases would open up a completely new mode of treating them. The success of this form of treatment would seem assured in view of Klenner's work on the viral diseases. The rickettsias should be just as vulnerable to ascorbic acid's action as the viruses. Clinical tests should be planned and started in these diseases without further delay.

McCormick (28), in 1951 and 1952, proposed the use of 2 to 4 grams of ascorbic acid, preferably by injection, in various infections. There are so many other papers reporting the use of ascorbic acid in various infections—in pharyngeal and eye infections (29), in brucellosis (a widespread disease) (30), in sinusitis (31), and a wide variety of other conditions; so many that it is impossible to cover them all adequately in the space of this chapter. In all the references cited in this chapter, except in a few isolated instances true megascorbic therapy was never used.

15

CANCER

Over half a million people in the United States develop cancer each year and over 280,000 will die of cancer in the year ahead. More than 700,000 people are under treatment at all times. It is the number two scourge and one of every five of us is likely to be afflicted; under present conditions it will send one of every eight of us to the grave.

Cancer is not a single disease entity but a large group of closely related, yet different, diseases. Essentially, cancerous growth is uncontrolled tissue development and expansion and is due to the tissue losing the normal restraints on cell division and growth. The cancer grows in a wild manner at the expense of the surrounding normal tissues. Cancer can arise in any organ or tissue of the body and, like the infectious diseases, the causes are varied and different. In severity it can range from a relatively innocuous minor illness to a life-threatening disease. The pattern of cancer incidence has been changing over the years, with fewer stomach and uterine cancers and more lung cancer and leukemia.

Present–Day Cancer Therapy

In the therapy of cancer, the first important step is diagnosis. After diagnosis, the physician has three different paths or a combination of them from which to choose: irradiation, chemotherapy, or surgery. Irradiation is localized exposure to X rays or to the radiant energy of radioactive sources, such as radium or cobalt 60, to try to kill the fast-growing cancerous tissue without doing too much damage to the rest of the body. Chemotherapy involves the use of chemical substances that tend to damage the cancer tissue more than the normal cells and thus retard the cancer development. Surgery, of course, is the direct approach of going in and physically removing the cancerous tissue, when possible.

Ever since the discovery of ascorbic acid in the early 1930s, there has been a vast amount of animal experimentation and clinical research conducted on the relationship of ascorbic acid to cancer. This has resulted in a mass of conflicting and confusing reports as to the value of ascorbic acid in cancer treatments. Some investigators reported good results in their tests, others reported no effects on the growth of cancer tissue, while still others took the stand that it stimulated tumor growth. Detailed discussion of the possible reasons for the conflicts of opinion in this work is beyond the scope of this chapter, except to speculate that it may be due to the wide variety of experimental animals, cancer types, and experimental conditions employed by the numerous investigators. As a first step in future cancer research on ascorbic acid, a responsible, unbiased research agency should review this large volume of early work and assess its value in the light of the more recent research and newer concepts. Any research work which may be required to resolve these unanswered questions and conflicting opinions should be conducted. Because of the long-standing disagreement and the resulting confusion, there has probably been a tendency for research workers to shy away from this area.

One thing, however, is certain. Cancer and its present-day therapy are intense biochemical stresses which deplete the bodies of cancer victims of their ascorbic acid. The irradiation, the surgery, or the chemotherapy with highly toxic materials, are all severe biochemical stresses. Biochemical stresses, in the majority of the mammals which are able to produce their own ascorbic acid, cause them to produce more ascorbic acid to combat the stresses. Because of their defective genetic inheritance, mammals such as guinea pigs, monkeys, and man are dependent on their food intake for ascorbic acid and their response to stress is ascorbic acid depletion.

Experiments on rats, mice, and guinea pigs are enlightening on this point. When rats and mice (animals that can make their own ascorbic acid) are exposed to cancer-producing agents (carcinogens), they start producing much more ascorbic acid in their livers (1). However, when guinea pigs (animals which, like man, cannot produce their own ascorbic acid) are exposed to the same carcinogens, their ascorbic acid is used up and not replaced (2); to quote the authors of this 1955 paper, when mammals are exposed to carcinogens this will "excite an increased demand for this compound (ascorbic acid) to which the animals capable of synthesizing it respond by overproduction, whereas in those lacking this power the store is depleted."

In another experiment on guinea pigs, Russell (3), in 1952, showed that cancers developed sooner in guinea pigs exposed to carcinogens and fed a diet deficient in ascorbic acid as compared to guinea pigs exposed to the same carcinogens but on an adequate ascorbic acid diet. Can we extrapolate this observation to humans and say that people who do not fully "correct" their genetic disease, hypoascorbemia, by continuously taking high levels of ascorbic acid are more susceptible to cancer than fully "corrected" individuals?

An opposite view is taken in the 1955 paper by Miller and Sokoloff (3), who proposed that a prescorbutic state in the cancer victim may have beneficial effects on cancer patients during radiation therapy. To settle this question once and for all should not entail much additional research. A person afflicted with cancer will almost always be nearly depleted of ascorbic acid before the usual course of therapy is begun. Radiation therapy using radiant energy in the form of X rays or gamma rays is a potent form of biochemical stress for the body. Exposing a cancer victim to radiant energy only further aggravates a serious shortage of this metabolite and prevents the body from maintaining biochemical homeostasis under the onslaughts of the additional radiation stresses. There have been other papers published which suggested giving ascorbic acid to cancer patients before exposure to radiation and noting its benefits (4). In spite of these many suggestions, further large-scale conclusive research has not been conducted and the practice is little used. These scientists, in their clinical work used, at most, a few grams of ascorbic acid a day. The full correction of the combined stresses of the cancer and the radiation may need much higher doses of ascorbic acid each day. This is another virgin area of megascorbic therapy, just awaiting someone to go in and try it.

Cancer chemotherapy is the use of certain chemicals to selectively poison the cancer cells without killing the patient. We will not go into the chemistry of the different materials used other than to say that they are all very poisonous and dangerous (host toxic). This, of course, limits the amounts which can be given the patient at any one time. One group of materials used in cancer chemotherapy is the so-called nitrogen mustards, which are derivatives of the mustard gases of World War I; you can conceive the type of material used in this therapy. While the chemotherapeutic agent will attack the cancer cells, the patient is left without means to overcome the toxic manifestations of the medicament. In spite of the fact that ascorbic acid has been known to be an efficient detoxicating agent for poisonous substances (see Chapter 24) no reports have been found in the medical literature for the combined administration of these toxic medicaments along with large doses of ascorbic acid as a supportive measure. The presence of high optimal levels of ascorbic acid might also improve the toxic action on the cancer cells (5), but we will never know unless it is thoroughly investigated. The potential benefits, if successful, would seem to make these clinical trials an urgent necessity.

The data contained in the 1969 paper from Dean Burk and his group (5) at the National Cancer Institute are very pertinent at this point. They showed that ascorbate is highly toxic to the cancer cells they used (Ehrlich ascites carcinoma cells) and caused profound structural changes in the cancer cells in their laboratory cultures. They mention that:

> The great advantage that ascorbates . . . possess as potential anticancer agents is that they are, like penicillin, remarkably nontoxic to normal body tissues, and they may be administered to animals in extremely large doses (up to 5 or more grams per kilogram) without notable harmful pharmacological effects.

5 grams per kilogram on a 70-kilogram adult would amount to 350 grams of ascorbic acid per day. They further state:

> In our view, the future of effective cancer chemotherapy will not rest on the use of host-toxic compounds now so widely employed, but upon virtually host-nontoxic compounds that are lethal to cancer cells, of which ascorbate . . . represents an excellent prototype example.

They also bring out the amazing fact that in the screening program that has been going on for years to find new cancer-killing materials at the Cancer Chemotherapy National Service Center, ascorbic acid has been bypassed, excluded from consideration, and never tested for its cancer-killing properties. The reason given for not screening ascorbic acid is even more fantastic—ascorbic acid was too nontoxic to fit into their program!

An almost immediate confirmation of Dean Burk's proposals was contained in the research conducted at Tulane University School of Medicine by Schlegel and coworkers and published in 1969 (5). It was shown that bladder cancer due to smoking and other causes could be prevented by ascorbic acid. They recommended the intake of 1.5 grams of ascorbic acid a day to avoid the recurrence of bladder tumors.

The remaining area of cancer therapy, surgery, is one where ascorbic acid may now be used to some extent. It may be used, not so much for its direct effect on the cancer, but for its beneficial effects in wound healing. For this purpose it is generally used at a gram or so a day, which may be quite inadequate to handle the biochemical stresses of anesthesia, surgical shock, and hemorrhagic shock on an already depleted cancer victim. Full "correction" of the victim's hypoascorbemia may require instituting a preoperative, operative, and postoperative regime at much higher levels. Additional research on a regime of this sort may uncover possibilities for survival and cure far beyond today's hopes.

Use of Ascorbic Acid in Cancer Therapy

Present-day cancer therapy thus virtually ignores the potential of ascorbic acid as a biochemical stress combatant, a detoxicant, an anticarcinogenic agent, a means for maintaining homeostasis, and a mechanism for improving the well-being and survival of the patient.

During the past forty years there have been many papers published in the medical literature in which ascorbic acid has been used for cancer therapy. But no one in all this time has consistently used ascorbic acid in the large doses which may be required to demonstrate a therapeutic effect. There has never been a well-planned program to test ascorbic acid in cancer therapy and no one has used more than a gram or, at most, several grams a day (except in one case, discussed later).

Deucher (4), in 1940, used up to 4 grams of ascorbic acid a day for several days in treating his cancer patients and found it had a

remarkably favorable effect on their general condition and increased their tolerance to X rays. On the other hand, Szenes (4), in
1942, stated that the administration of ascorbic acid is contraindi-
cated in tumor patients because it intensifies tumor growth.

It was also used in combination with vitamin A, which only
further complicated the picture, in a series of tests. Von Wendt, in
1949, 1950, and 1951, and Huber, in 1953, used 2 grams of
ascorbic acid a day combined with large doses of vitamin A and
reported favorable effects. Schneider, in 1954, 1955, and 1956,
also used ascorbic acid, 1 gram daily in combination with vitamin
A, and found that it "arrested" cancers and that it was more useful
against epitheliomas than against sarcomas (6).

Of interest also are three papers by McCormick (7), in 1954,
1959, and 1963, in which he postulates the theory that the factor
which preconditions the body to the development of cancer is the
degenerative changes caused by continued low levels of ascorbic
acid in the body. He gives evidence to support his hypothesis and
states, "We maintain that the degree of malignancy is determined
inversely by the degree of connective tissue resistance, which in
turn is dependent upon the adequacy of vitamin C status." McCormick's ideas have never been adequately tested.

Some additional evidence for the support of this hypothesis
comes from the work of Goth and Littmann (8), in 1948, who
found that cancers most frequently originate in organs whose ascorbic acid levels are below 4.5 mg % and rarely grow in organs
containing ascorbic acid above this concentration. Fully corrected
individuals should have tissue levels of ascorbic acid in excess of
this seemingly critical 4.5 mg %.

Detoxication of Carcinogens

Another piece of research which has not been properly followed
through was reported by Warren (9), in 1943, who showed that
certain carcinogens, anthracene, and 3:4-benzpyrene (the type of
carcinogen in tobacco smoke), are susceptible to oxidation in the
presence of ascorbic acid. In the oxidized form they are no longer
carcinogenic.

Here is a possible means for preventing the induction of cancer
after exposure to carcinogens merely by maintaining the necessary
levels of ascorbic acid in the exposed tissues. This is an area of
research that has been stagnant for two decades, which would have

the most important consequences for smokers or city dwellers forced to breathe polluted air, or for others exposed to carcinogens.

Leukemia

Leukemia is a cancerous disease of the blood-forming tissues in which there is an overproduction of the white blood cells (leukocytes). Different types of leukemia are named after the different varieties of leukocytes involved in the disease process. The overproduction of the leukocytes causes, in most cases, a marked rise in the numbers of white blood cells in the circulating blood.

Research work connecting ascorbic acid, the blood elements, and leukemia was started not long after the discovery of ascorbic acid. Stephen and Hawley (10), in 1936, showed that when the blood was separated into plasma, red blood cells, and white blood cells, there was a 20- to 30-fold concentration of ascorbic acid in the white blood cells.

Hemorrhage, being a symptom of both leukemia and scurvy, caused clinicians to early investigate the use of ascorbic acid in leukemia because of its dramatic effects on hemorrhage in scurvy. Eufinger and Gaehtgens (11), in 1936, reported giving 200 milligrams of ascorbic acid a day and came to the conclusion that it had a normalizing influence on the blood picture. Schnetz (11), in 1940, came to the same conclusion: when the leukocytes are high ascorbic acid tends to reduce them, and when they are low it tends to increase them. He used 200 to 900 milligrams a day by injection.

Here is a marked example of the ancient mammalian mechanism of ascorbic acid homeostasis.

In 1936, Plum and Thomsen (12), injecting 200 milligrams of ascorbic acid a day, obtained remissions in two cases of myeloid leukemia, and Heinild and Schiedt (12), using two 100-milligram injections daily, obtained uncertain, variable results. Thiele (12), in 1938, using 500 milligrams of ascorbic acid a day by injection, found no effect in chronic myeloid leukemia, while both Palenque (4) and van Nieuwenhuizen (12), in 1943, observed slight decreases in the white blood counts. Such variable and confusing results are typical when submarginal and inadequate dosages are employed.

Vogt, in 1940, in a review of the work conducted on ascorbic acid in leukemia up to that time, cited twenty-one references.

About the only conclusion he reached was that there were high deficits of ascorbic acid in leukemics. These deficits and the very low blood plasma levels of ascorbic acid in leukemics were confirmed in later papers by Kyhos et al., in 1945, and Waldo and Zipf, in 1955, and yet, in all these years, no one was inspired to get away from these pitifully small doses of ascorbic acid and make some clinical tests with heroic doses (13).

In a leukemic, the biochemical stresses of the disease process has reduced the body stores of ascorbic acid to very low levels. Any ascorbic acid circulating in the blood has been scavenged and locked in the excessive numbers of white blood cells contained in the blood. The plasma level of ascorbic acid is usually zero or close thereto. A zero level in the blood plasma means that the tissues of the body are not being supplied with this most important metabolite. The ascorbic acid contained in the leukocytes are unavailable for the tissues. The tissues are in a condition of biochemical scurvy and this explains why these depleted tissues are so susceptible to the characteristic hemorrhaging of leukemia and the infections that kill so many of the leukemics. A leukemic is not only suffering from leukemia but also from a bad case of biochemical scurvy. To correct this condition, ascorbic acid has to be administered in sufficiently large doses not only to saturate the excess of white blood cells but to provide adequate spillover into the blood plasma and tissues so that the seriously ill leukemic will be given a fighting chance to combat the disease. This may require the administration of ascorbic acid at the rate of 25 or more grams per day, as noted in the following case of leukemia treated with megascorbic levels of ascorbic acid.

This case history, reported by Greer (14), in 1954, was of a seventy-one-year-old executive of an oil company, who was first seen for alcoholic cirrhosis of the liver and polycythemia (excess of red blood cells); some months earlier, symptoms of chronic myocarditis had appeared. Shortly thereafter, he was hospitalized and passed a large uric acid bladder stone, and a diagnosis of chronic myelogenous leukemia was established. He also had intractable pyorrhea and his remaining 17 teeth were removed at one operation. At this time he started taking ascorbic acid at the rate of 24.5 grams to 42 grams per day, "because he reported he felt much better when he took these large doses." Since the diagnosis of leukemia and the removal of the teeth, "the patient has repeatedly remarked about his feeling of well-being and has continued his vocation as executive of an oil company." On two occasions, at the insistence of his attending physician, he stopped taking the ascorbic acid and both times his spleen and liver enlarged and became tender, his temperature rose to 101°, and he complained of general malaise and fatigue (typical leukemia symptoms). When he started the ascorbic acid again, the symptoms cleared and his temperature became normal within 6 hours. Over a year and a half later the patient had a severe attack of epidemic diarrhea and died of acute cardiac decompensation. At the time of death, the spleen was firm, not tender, and had not enlarged since taking the ascorbic acid. The doctor also reported that "the polycythemia, leukemia, cirrhosis, and the myocarditis had shown no progression" in the year and a half while taking the ascorbic acid. The case history concludes with the statement, "The intake of the huge doses of ascorbic acid appeared essential for the welfare of the patient."

One would believe that the exciting results in this 1954 case would be immediately picked up and explored further by the leukemia groups in the national government or the foundations that are continually asking the public for more research money, but no follow-up work has been found in the medical literature of the past sixteen years. If megascorbic therapy could do so much for an aged leukemic with so many other complications, what could it do for the young, uncomplicated leukemic? The answer to this question could be obtained easily and each day lost may mean more lives wasted. At the present time, millions of dollars are spent in screening all sorts of poisonous chemicals for use in leukemia, while a harmless substance like ascorbic acid, with so much potential, lies around neglected and ignored.

Recent work has brought forward evidence that human leukemia may be caused by a virus. While viruses are known to produce cancerlike diseases in animals, none have been proved in man. If the cause of human leukemia is eventually shown to be due to a virus, the rationale for the use of megascorbic therapy in leukemia will be further strengthened because it has been shown that ascorbic acid is a potent, wide-spectrum, nontoxic virucide when used at megascorbic dosage levels (see Chapter 13).

16

THE HEART, VASCULAR SYSTEM, AND STROKES

The diseases of the heart and the cardiovascular system are the number one killers of present-day Americans. The reported incidence of these diseases has been rising sharply. A few years ago heart diseases accounted for over 700,000 deaths annually and strokes took another 200,000. The number of cardiovascular deaths among persons under sixty-five (about 240,000) was about as high as deaths from cancer at all ages. Besides death, heart diseases cause widespread illness and disability and impose a multi-billion-dollar burden on the economy each year. In a recent health survey, it was found that of every hundred persons between the ages of eighteen and seventy-nine, thirteen had definite heart disease and twelve more were suspect. Nearly one-quarter of the population, therefore, lives in jeopardy of succumbing to a disease of the heart or circulatory system. The incidence increases with age.

Because our cardiovascular system is so important, let us first look into the equipment with which we are endowed. We have a complicated plumbing arrangement comprising a closed system of interconnected flexible pipes. The system has a dual pumping arrangement combined in one hard-working organ, the heart. The flexible arteries carrying the blood, under pressure, away from the pump are the largest, and subdivide into smaller and smaller vessels until those carrying the blood into the tissues, the capillaries, are microscopic in size. The blood in the tissues is then collected in flexible vessels of increasing diameter, the venules and veins, for its trip back to the pump for another strong push into the arteries. This process goes on twenty-four hours a day for the entire lifetime of the individual.

The pump and the flexible pipes in this system must be rugged to start with and must be in a constant state of self-repair and maintenance to withstand the continual wear and tear of the alternating mechanical stresses of fluid flow. Should any structural weakness in the walls occur or leaks develop anywhere in the closed system, we are in serious trouble with heart disease, strokes, and hemorrhaging.

The main structural element, from which this system is built and which provides the strength, elasticity, and ruggedness is the protein collagen. This protein comprises about one-third of the body's protein content and is the cement substance which holds the tissues and organs together. The synthesis of collagen by the body requires the presence of ascorbic acid. Without ascorbic acid, collagen cannot be produced. If too little ascorbic acid is present during the synthesis of collagen, it will be defective and structurally weak. Ascorbic acid is also required for the maintenance of the integrity of the collagen already synthesized in the continuing process of self-repair and self-maintenance of the tissues and the vascular system.

It is necessary, therefore, to have sufficient ascorbic acid available during fetal life to provide structurally sound collagen for the development of the cardiovascular system and to have sufficient ascorbic acid available during the entire lifetime of the individual to maintain this collagen in the proper state of self-repair. Impaired and structurally weak collagen is the cause of the most distressing symptoms of uncorrected hypoascorbemia (clinical scurvy), the scorbutic bleeding gums, the loose teeth, the capillary bleeding, the reopening of old healed wounds and scars, and the brittle bones. Most of our mammalian relatives, whose livers are continually producing large amounts of ascorbic acid, need never worry about this because they do not develop scurvy.

It is the author's belief that the high incidence of cardio-vascular disease in man is brought on because the greater part of the human population is dependent upon their foodstuffs as a source for their ascorbic acid intake and are thus existing on submarginal levels. These intakes are usually inadequate for the production and maintenance of optimal high-strength collagen over long periods of time. Because the system is subjected to many local ascorbic acid-depleting stresses, an abundant supply of ascorbic acid is demanded, not just "vitamin" levels.

Shortly after the discovery of ascorbic acid in the early 1930s, the intimate association of it with the cardiovascular system was surmised. This resulted in a tremendous amount of research and a considerable body of medical literature.

In 1934, Rinehart and Mettier (1) found that infected guinea pigs deprived of ascorbic acid developed degenerative lesions of the heart valves and muscles. The changes were strikingly similar to those seen in rheumatic fever. Infected guinea pigs maintained with adequate ascorbic acid did not develop these heart lesions. A year later, Menten and King (2) injected sublethal doses of diphtheria toxin into ascorbic acid-deficient guinea pigs and produced myocardial degeneration and arteriosclerosis of the lungs, liver, spleen, and kidneys. In further tests on guinea pigs with acute or chronic scurvy (3), it was indicated they developed inflammation of their heart valves, myocarditis, and occasional pericarditis.

As early as 1941 (4), it was suspected that inadequate intake of ascorbic acid was a factor in coronary thrombosis due to impaired collagen production, causing capillary rupture and hemorrhage in the arterial walls. Blood plasma ascorbic acid measurements were made in 455 consecutive adult patients admitted to the Ottawa Civic Hospital over a seven-month period and it was found that 56 percent had subnormal levels (below 0.5 mg %) and 81 percent of the coronary patients were in this subnormal range. It was "recommended that patients with coronary artery disease be assured of an adequate vitamin C (ascorbic acid) intake." A 1947 paper (5) showed that inadequate ascorbic acid body levels were not limited to cardiac patients of the lower economic brackets. The survey included 556 private patients, of which 123 had organic heart disease. Forty-two percent of all patients, 59 percent of the heart patients, and 70 percent of the coronary thrombotic patients had low plasma levels of ascorbic acid (below 0.5 mg %). Sixty-five percent of the coronary group had dangerously low levels (0.35 mg % or less). Again it was suggested that ascorbic acid be used as an adjunct to the usual methods of treatment, especially in the long-range care in the postinfarctive period.

A provocative series of papers was published by Dr. G. C. Willis and coworkers starting in 1953 that showed the importance of ascorbic acid in the maintenance of the integrity of the arterial walls (the intima). Any factor disturbing ascorbic acid metabolism, either systemically or locally, results in wall injury with subsequent fatlike deposits. In his 1953 paper, Willis (6) concludes that acute or chronic ascorbic acid deficiency in guinea pigs produces atherosclerosis and closely simulates the human form of the disease. Cholesterol feeding interferes with the ascorbic acid metabolism of rabbits and guinea pigs and intraperitoneal injection of ascorbic acid inhibits the atherosclerosis in cholesterol-fed guinea pigs. Finally he states, "Massive doses of parenteral ascorbic acid may be of therapeutic value in the treatment of atherosclerosis and the prevention of intimal hemorrhage and thrombosis." In 1954, the Willis group (7) studied the actual progression and regression of atherosclerotic plaques in living patients by a serial X-ray technique. Both progression and regression were observed over relatively short periods of time but did not coexist in the same cases during one period of observation. The rationale for ascorbic acid therapy is again outlined and preliminary results of such therapy were encouraging. In 1955, there appeared another paper (8), in which scientists actually examined the ascorbic acid levels in the fresh arteries from cases of sudden death, hospital autopsy material, and cases treated with ascorbic acid for various lengths of time before death. The conclusions reached in this study are so exciting and important that they are quoted in full:

1. A gross and often complete deficiency of ascorbic acid frequently exists in the arteries of apparently well-nourished hospital autopsy subjects. Old age seems to accentuate the deficiency.
2. The ascorbic acid depletion is probably not nutritional but rather related to the stress of the fatal illness.
3. A localized depletion often exists in segments of arteries

susceptible to atherosclerosis for reasons of mechanical stress. Adjacent segments, whose mechanical stress is less, tend to have a higher ascorbic acid content and atherosclerosis here is rare.

4. The significance of this ascorbic acid depletion lies in the fact that scurvy in guinea pigs results in the rapid onset of atherosclerosis. Furthermore it has been reported that the aorta can synthesize cholesterol and the incorporation of radioactive acetate into cholesterol in tissues is said to be several times more rapid in tissues depleted of ascorbic acid.

5. Ascorbic acid deficiency in arteries with resulting ground substance depolymerization may account for the release of glucoprotein noted in the blood of subjects with severe atherosclerosis.

6. Preliminary studies suggest that it is possible to replenish the ascorbic acid in arteries by ascorbic acid therapy.

A similar concept was proposed, in 1957, by McCormick (9), noting the importance of ascorbic acid deficiency in coronary thrombosis. He summarized his work as follows:

Thrombosis is not in itself a pernicious development but rather a protective response of the organism designed normally to effect repair of damaged blood vessels by cicatrization. High blood pressure, excessive stretching of blood vessels and deficiency of (ascorbic acid) vitamin C, resulting in rupture and bleeding of the intima at the site of such stress initiate the development of the thrombosis by means of the clotting of the blood, which is also a protective reaction. This multiple protective mechanism should be sustained and controlled by physiological means (vitamin C therapy) rather than suppressed by anticoagulants with their dangerous side effects.

McCormick believed that an optimal body level of ascorbic acid offered the best natural means of effecting healthy new tissue, and claims that the initial intimal hemorrhage, precipitating thrombosis, would not occur if adequate prophylactic use of ascorbic acid were made to maintain the integrity of the cardiovascular system.

There is an extensive body of published research showing the intimate relationship between ascorbic acid and cholesterol metabolisms. In fact, the published research on the subject of the relationship of ascorbic acid to heart disease is so extensive that it is quite impossible to review it adequately and still keep within the bounds of a reasonable size for this chapter.

Cholesterol was identified as a major constituent of the arterial deposit over a century ago (10). As early as 1913 it was demonstrated that feeding cholesterol to rabbits resulted in atheromatous deposits in their aortas (11). In 1953, an intimate relationship between ascorbic acid and the synthesis of cholesterol in guinea pigs was shown by C. G. King and his group (12). Ascorbic acid deprivation greatly increased cholesterol synthesis. This observation was confirmed on guinea pigs fed an atherogenic diet (13). This group found that the greater the deprivation of ascorbic acid, the more the cholesterol accumulated in the tissues. The feeding of cholesterol to rabbits and guinea pigs lowers ascorbic acid levels (14) in the body, and coronary atherosclerosis appears to be in part a possible result of deficient ingestion of ascorbic acid (15). Increased intakes of ascorbic acid bring down cholesterol levels in rabbits (16), guinea pigs (17), rats (18), and humans (19).

Further confirmation of the ability of ascorbic acid to reduce cholesterol levels was reported in 1971 by R. O. Mumma and coworkers (20) and C. R. Spittle (20). Ascorbic acid sulfate was found to be a significant metabolite of ascorbic acid in human urine by E. M. Baker III and coworkers in 1971 (20). Spittle observed that the blood serum levels of cholesterol could be varied by changing the ascorbic acid intake. She suggested "that atherosclerosis is a long-term deficiency (or negative balance) of vitamin C which permits cholesterol levels to build up in the arterial system and results in changes in other fractions of the fats."

A most exciting paper by G. C. Willis (20) appeared in 1957 entitled "The Reversibility of Atherosclerosis." In this study atherosclerosis was induced in guinea pigs by depriving them of ascorbic acid. Some guinea pigs were then given large doses of ascorbic acid and it was found that in these animals the beginning atherosclerotic lesions were rapidly resorbed while the more advanced atherosclerotic plaques on the artery walls took longer. There was a steady decline in the incidence of the lesions in direct proportion to the duration of ascorbic acid therapy. The significance of these observations for man is tremendous—they open the way to the megascorbic prophylaxis of atherosclerosis—but they never were tested further.

Naturally occurring arteriosclerosis is found in many different mammals besides man. A recent study (21) showed there is a pronounced difference between atherosclerotic disease in various mammals as compared to various primates, including man. Fatty deposits play a relatively minor role in the naturally occurring lesions observed in the coronary arteries of the dog, cat, elephant, and other lower animals. In some of these animals there seems to be virtually no lipid involvement in the diseased arteries. In the primates, lipid deposition in the arteriosclerotic lesion is more pronounced, and distinct atherosclerotic plaques develop in man. The most significant physiological difference between the dog, cat, elephant, and other lower animals and the group of primates studied and man is that the former group of mammals are able to produce ascorbic acid in their livers in large daily amounts while the primates used in this investigation and man cannot do this. This is just another pertinent observation on the importance of this synthetic liver-enzyme system for the mammals and the vital involvement of ascorbic acid in the genesis of atherosclerosis. A similar observation was made in 1962 (22) regarding the response of rats and guinea pigs to the development of atherosclerosis. Rats are known to be resistant to atherosclerotic changes, while guinea pigs are not. Here again the difference between these two species is that the rat is a good producer of ascorbic acid in its liver while the guinea pig, like man, is genetically unable to do so.

Another property of ascorbic acid that has been neglected in the treatment of the edema of heart disease is its diuretic properties at high dosage levels. Abnormal retention of water throughout the body was noted in the post mortem examination by Lind in 1753 of patients dying of scurvy. Soon after the discovery of ascorbic acid in 1936 and 1937 (23), its diuretic properties were recognized in spite of the small doses of ascorbic acid employed. Its use in heart failure was suggested in 1938 by Evans (24), who pointed out the need for "an adequate supply of vitamin C for all patients with heart failure." Other papers in the period from 1944 to 1952 indicated its diuretic usefulness (25). Still, even at the present time, it is not being used. In intensive care units for coronaries, ascorbic acid is conspicuous by its absence.

Cerebrovascular Accidents — Strokes

Over 200,000 deaths occur annually from strokes, and another 800,000 persons are totally or partially disabled by them. Major brain hemorrhages or thrombosis account for the sudden demise or total disablement. But of even greater incidence is the slow destruction of neural tissues of the brain by repetitive, small local thrombosis, or capillary rupture, with intimal hemorrhage (little strokes). It has been estimated that there are at least 1,200,000 people in the United States who have suffered one or more of these little strokes. They happen, and most of the time pass unnoticed, with nothing more to indicate their passing than a slight dizziness or nausea. It is only when the summation of these minor brain injuries cause mental or physical deterioriation, to a point where it is noticeable by the patient or the family, that it becomes evident that something is wrong. By that time, it is too late to do anything about it. What is needed is a prophylactic regime to prevent this situation and forestall little strokes.

In order to maintain the integrity of the vascular system of the brain, ascorbic acid is needed, as it is in any other part of the body except more so. The brain itself requires much ascorbic acid for its own active metabolism and functioning, so if one is completely dependent on the submarginal levels of ascorbic acid supplied by foodstuffs, asymptomatic chronic vascular damage results which only becomes evident when a major part gives way and massive hemorrhages or thrombi develop. Suboptimal levels of ascorbic acid not only lead to strokes, but when fresh brain tissue from autopsies on patients dying of cerebral vascular disorders were examined, ascorbic acid was found to be entirely lacking or at extremely low, subnormal levels (26). In a four-year study on the continuous administration of varying amounts of ascorbic acid to thirty-two elderly patients with vascular disease, Gale and Thewlis (27), in 1953, reported six deaths. Four were directly due to heart attacks or cerebral episodes. Of these four, not one had taken more than the low level of 100 milligrams of ascorbic acid daily during the test period. They stated:

> Many symptoms of vascular disturbances in the aged suggest that latent scurvy may be a frequent occurrence. . . . Extended studies should be made by public health departments and geriatric clinics to determine the effectiveness of vitamins C and P in controlling cardiac and cerebrovascular illness.

How often do we hear this refrain, and yet nothing is ever done?

In spite of the dire need to do something effective in the prevention and therapy of this terrible plague of cardiovascular disease and cerebrovascular episodes, all this provocative and suggestive research has been glossed over and ignored and none of the crucial large-scale tests have ever been made. One possible excuse for this neglect might be that nearly all of the work was done by researchers whose viewpoint was clouded by the narrow confines of the vitamin C hypothesis and who had used inadequate dosage levels of ascorbic acid for maximal therapeutic effects. This should no longer be the case, for the description of the genetic disease hypoascorbemia in man (28) supplies the needed rationale for the megascorbic prophylactic doses which may be required to reduce the incidence of heart disease and for the megascorbic therapeutic doses which may be required to treat heart disease when it occurs.

The crucial tests would include taking a large population of individuals and administering continued long-term (for the rest of their lifetime) megascorbic prophylactic levels of ascorbic acid (about 70 milligrams per kilogram of body weight per day, or about 3 to 5 grams a day in spaced doses for an adult) and then measure the incidence and morbidity of disease at intervals and the increase in healthy lifespan as compared to a similar population on placebos. For heart disease therapy, we need to try megascorbic therapy in emergency coronary care units using doses of possibly 1,000 milligrams per kilogram of body weight per day, intravenously at first, and then working out a dosage schedule as the patient comes out of danger. Similarly, in cerebrovascular accident treatments, megascorbic therapy may introduce a new era in post-episode survival and recovery, and prevention of future strokes by the mere elimination of the localized cerebral scurvy that exists in stroke victims.

All of this provocative and suggestive research, conducted all over the world for the last four decades, indicates that the simple ingestion of 3 to 5 grams of ascorbic acid a day in several spaced doses may be sufficient as a megascorbic prophylactic regime to prevent the high incidence of heart disease and strokes. The potential victims of these diseases may live a healthier life far beyond the time when these diseases would be cutting them down. In acute cases of massive coronary or cerebral hemorrhage, the prompt application of megascorbic therapy in intensive care units would seem to assure survival to those now destined to die because of their severe, uncorrected hypoascorbemia.

17

ARTHRITIS AND RHEUMATISM

Approximately 13 million Americans suffer from arthritis, making it the nation's number-one crippler. Over 10 million have seen a doctor seeking relief and more than 3 million report limitation of their usual activity because of the disease. An estimated 1.3 billion dollars is the yearly toll on the economy (1).

Arthritis is not a killing disease, so the prevalence rises with age, the victims becoming disabled and wracked with pain—but they continue to live and suffer. Arthritis gradually withdraws from productive activity large numbers of otherwise capable people.

Arthritis, rheumatism, and other related conditions are often referred to as the collagen diseases because of the definite involvement of this protein in their genesis and cause. Anyone having read the previous chapter on heart disease will recall the relation of ascorbic acid to collagen production and the absolute necessity for the presence of high levels of ascorbic acid in the body for the proper synthesis and maintenance of high-quality collagen protein. Briefly, collagen makes up about a third of our body's protein content. It is the deprivation of ascorbic acid, with the consequent synthesis of poor quality collagen or no synthesis at all, which brings on the most distressing bone and joint effects of clinical scurvy. There can be no doubt about the intimate association of ascorbic acid and the collagen diseases.

Rivers (2), in 1965, in a review article on the tissue derangements caused by a lack of ascorbic acid states, "Abnormalities in this protein (collagen) are basic to the crippling deformities associated with rheumatic diseases and with a number of congenital connective tissue defects." Robertson (3), in studies on induced granuloma tissue of prescorbutic and normal guinea pigs, showed that guinea pigs deprived of ascorbic acid for only 14 days produced tissue containing only 2 to 3 percent collagen, while the tissues in normal guinea pigs contain 14 to 16 percent. Udenfriend (4), Stone and Meister (5), and many others have shown that the dependence of high-quality collagen protein on ascorbic acid is due to its chemical action on one or two of the amino acid building blocks used in the manufacture of collagen.

As in many other diseases, the discovery of ascorbic acid inspired much research on the collagen diseases in the 1930s. A classic series of papers by Rinehart and coworkers (6) appeared in the period from 1933 to 1938 relating deficiencies of ascorbic acid and infection to the development of the rheumatoid process. They developed a theory intimately linking ascorbic acid with the genesis of rheumatic fever from the evidence of its social, urban, and familial incidence, the role of malnutrition, the age of incidence, seasonal incidence, geographic distribution, the symptomatic similarities of latent scurvy with the early rheumatic state, the role of infection, the problems of hemorrhage, and the existence of latent scurvy in rheumatics. Their logic was impeccable and everything fitted together like a jigsaw puzzle. They then confirmed these postulates by experimentally producing rheumatoid lesions in the guinea pig by combining ascorbic acid deprivation and infection. Infection alone did not produce these effects. It seemed that here, at last, was the answer to the age-old problem of the rheumatic diseases.

As might be expected, the publication of Rinehart's series of papers evoked much discussion and further tests. The papers resulting from this additional work may be divided into those that agreed with and more or less checked Rhinehart's work (7) and those that disagreed (8). Reviewing these discussions in detail now would serve no useful purpose and would occupy too much space.

If anyone is interested, they can refer to the original papers. Of vital importance is the clinical work conducted, in these early days, to test Rinehart's hypotheses; and we shall see with the advantage of hindsight how this clinical work was inadequate. We will first review the clinical work on dosages at the "vitamin" levels and observe their general ineffectiveness. After this we will take up the scant clinical data where tests were conducted using ascorbic acid at the lower fringes of megascorbic therapy with good clinical results.

M. P. Schultz (9), in 1936, reported on tests conducted at the hospital of the Rockefeller Institute in which ambulatory patients received from 100 to 250 milligrams of ascorbic acid daily either orally or intravenously for periods of months (the average was 2½ months). The conclusion was that the incidence of rheumatic fever or the clinical manifestations of the disease were not favorably or demonstrably affected by this medication. F. H. Mosse (10), in 1938, described a single case, the dramatic improvement of a farmer with acute multiple arthritis, in the midst of a scurvy epidemic in China, by the ingestion of 800 to 1200 cubic centimeters of "fresh red fruit juice." He also discussed the etiology of rheumatic fever in northern China in those days. M. G. Hall and coworkers (11) at the P. B. Brigham Hospital in Boston reported, in 1939, that all of the patients with rheumatoid arthritis were placed on an intake of 200 milligrams of ascorbic acid per day for eight months with no improvement that could be attributed to this treatment.

In 1940, R. H. Jacques (12) reported that in a series of forty-eight arthritic cases, forty-seven had low levels of ascorbic acid in their blood plasma. Treatment with 100 milligrams a day of injectable ascorbic acid for one week and 300 milligrams a day of ascorbic acid orally for another few weeks brought up the blood plasma levels. The patients were followed for a period of three weeks to six months thereafter on a regime of 100 milligrams of ascorbic acid a day orally. His conclusion—there was no marked clinical response even though the plasma levels had returned to normal. Twenty percent were moderately improved, 33 percent were slightly improved, and 47 percent showed no change or were worse. In a short report in a Russian journal, Vilyansky (13) treated thirty-nine patients with 200 to 300 milligrams of ascorbic acid intravenously per day. He reported that his tests showed his patients to be quite deficient in ascorbic acid and they responded well to the treatment. There was less pain, better mood, less swelling, and increased mobility in twenty-six of his patients. Eleven took longer to respond and two showed no effect. These two had been treated previously with salicylates. He states that in most cases three to five injections of ascorbic acid were sufficient to "liquidate" the attack of rheumatism.

Freyberg (14), in 1942, using fruit juices or ascorbic acid in amounts to maintain the blood plasma levels at "normal" levels in thirty-seven patients, found that "there was no evidence that the arthritis was better or that the course of the disease was different in any way whether or not the vitamin C deficiency was corrected." Trant and Matousek (15), in 1949, reported their experiences treating a series of eighteen arthritic patients at Chicago Presbyterian Hospital with 100 milligrams of ascorbic acid daily. They concluded, "On the principle of good hygiene it is well to restore low levels of serum ascorbic acid to normal, but not with the anticipation that any improvement in the arthritis will result."

Rinehart (16), in 1943, in a paper entitled "Rheumatic Fever and Nutrition," reviewed the work of the previous decade and admitted:

> While it has been shown that vitamin C does not exert a specific curative effect upon rheumatic fever it is likely that the frequency and severity of the hemorrhagic manifestations have been reduced. It is not known to what extent vitamin C or related factors might further protect the patient. Maintenance of rheumatic patients on adequate amounts of ascorbic acid will evidently not prevent recurrence of the disease.

The conclusions to be drawn from these early tests are that the measurement of ascorbic acid blood levels is not a good criterion for therapeutic effects and that the approach used by all these investigators was wrong. They were trying to correct a nutritional deficiency instead of treating a serious disease. The daily dosages required to raise the blood levels of ascorbic acid to what they considered normal were greatly below the megascorbic levels actually required to obtain a definite therapeutic effect in the collagen diseases. These early clinical tests were experiments in home economics rather than the thorough pharmacological testing of a new medicament.

Massell (17), in 1950, in a preliminary report on the use of 4 grams of ascorbic acid (1 gram four times per day) in seven young patients (five to eighteen years) for only eight to twenty-six days obtained rapid cessation of symptoms and stated, "Our observations suggest that ascorbic acid when administered in sufficient amounts possesses antirheumatic activity." He also mentions:

> Previous therapeutic failure may perhaps be attributed to the fact that practically all investigators were thinking in terms of vitamin C deficiency and, hence, used doses of ascorbic acid considerably smaller than those used by us. . . . It is possible that individual doses of more than 1 gram or total daily doses of more than 4 grams, if found harmless, may prove to be therapeutically even more effective.

The purpose of the publication of this preliminary report was to "stimulate further investigations of the therapeutic potentialities of ascorbic acid." Large-scale tests were never made to check these exciting results. The only further testings which were made are the following highly successful clinical tests reported in the 1950s by private investigators—then we have silence.

Baufeld (18), in 1952, using individual intravenous dosages of 6 grams of ascorbic acid for acute and chronic rheumatism, observed "astonishing" results in some cases. He also noticed good response in lumbago, sciatica, and bronchial asthma. He stated that he believed he had found something which called for further testing. In 1953, Greer (19) found 8 to 12 grams of ascorbic acid, in combination with antibiotics, to be an effective antirheumatic fever measure in several serious cases. McCormick (20), in 1955, after offering a scholarly review of the literature dating back to the seventeenth century, showed the relationship of scurvy to the rheumatic diseases and stated that a number of his acute rheumatic fever cases were treated with 1 to 10 grams of ascorbic acid daily with a rapid and complete recovery in three to four weeks without cardiac complications. Similar results were obtained in incipient arthritis. Afanasieva (21), in a 1959 Russian paper, noted gains in 48 rheumatic fever women patients using 1.25 grams of ascorbic acid daily for twenty to twenty-five days in combination with other therapy.

If the government agencies and the publicly supported foundations interested in the arthritic diseases, had pursued these scant but provocative leads supplied by Massell and others in the 1950s, the past two decades may have seen the elimination of these collagen diseases as a major crippler of the population.

18

AGING

If the aging process is looked upon as a chronic, 100 percent fatal disease from which everyone suffers and which is present at birth and continues with increasing ferocity throughout life, we have a logical viewpoint to start our discussion. The first conclusion we can draw is that treatment of this chronic disease should not be directed against the acute symptoms developing in the later years but should be in prophylactic, preventive measures starting at birth and continuing throughout life.

Further, if we look at some statistics on the human life span, we find some startling facts. Modern medicine can take credit for the rise in *life expectancy at birth* of nearly twenty years from the 49.2 years in 1900 and much more from earlier days (it was 38.7 in 1840). This stems from the drop in infant mortality and reduction of morbidity of childhood diseases. But, as pointed out by Bjorksten (1), in 1965, the life expectancy for those at age sixty has been practically the same since 1789 (Figure 4). Medicine has not done much to prolong the life span for those who survive the early hazardous years.

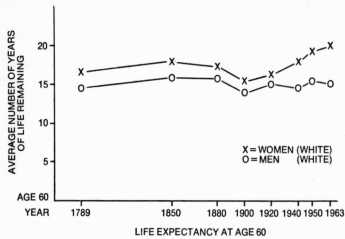

Figure 4.

From *Vital Statistics of the United States,*
1963, Vol. II, Section 5, Life Table 5-5

COMPARISON OF PRESENT MORTALITY CURVE WITH PROJECTED
CURVES BEFORE AND AFTER A BREAKTHROUGH IN GERIATRIC RESEARCH

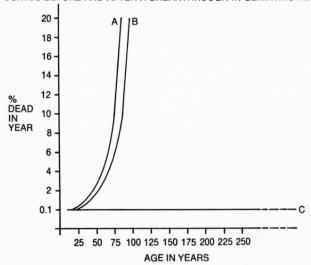

A. Present mortality curve (U.S. Bureau of Census). B. Estimated mortality curve,
if heart and other circulatory diseases, cancer, renal, and respiratory diseases were
eliminated, but no progress were made on aging. C. Mortality curve, if no further
progress were made on any specific disease, but the progressive loss of resistance
due to aging were eliminated. (Bjorksten, 1965)

Figure 5

Bjorksten (1), in 1963, also compared the present mortality curves with a projected line which would be obtained if medical research were able to eliminate the progressive loss of resistance due to aging. The line was stopped at age 300 because there was no more room on the graph.

It was also recently noted by this author (2) that the current statistics on the human life span do not give a true picture of potential longevity because the "normal" population (which would be represented by lines A and B in Figure 5) used in the calculation of these statistics was suffering from uncorrected hypoascorbemia. Statistics based on a population of fully corrected individuals could be entirely different. The importance of the proper synthesis and maintenance of the vital protein, collagen, as a prime factor in inhibiting aging was also indicated. This synthesis and maintenance is wholly dependent on ascorbic acid.

The author believes that it is now practical to travel along line C of Figure 5 by the full "correction" of the genetic disease, hypoascorbemia, throughout life. The only tests needed are to see how far along line C we can travel. It is also his opinion that the proper use of ascorbic acid *throughout* life may provide the long-awaited breakthrough in geriatrics. Perhaps most importantly, ascorbic acid should also *prolong the period of vigorous and healthy maturity,* not merely prolong the life span.

The current theories relating to aging are backed by a substantial volume of published papers of which we can cite only a few. The work of F. Verzár, W. Reichel, F. M. Sinex, D. Harman, I. G. Fels, and J. Bjorksten (1, 3) indicates that senescence is due to profound changes in the elastic and other properties of the various tissue macromolecules. These changes are provoked by various environmental factors such as oxidation, free radicals, radiation, cross-linking, stress, and others, combined with time. Their research indicates that collagen is a very important factor in the aging process.

Here we are back again on the collagen-track with all the implications of the basic involvement of ascorbic acid in maintaining the collagen molecules in good repair and "young."

Many other reports of tests on the aging of the collagen macromolecule have confirmed the suspicion of its direct involvement in aging (4) (F. M. Sinex, 1957; A. Aslan and A. Vrabiesco, 1965; F. Verzár and H. Spichtin, 1966; C. D. Nordschow, 1966; R.

Goodman, 1970, and many others). The extensive bibliographies given in these published reports indicate the vast amount of research expended in this field.

The use of antioxidants has been suggested many times to counteract the cross-linking and aggregative effects of oxidation and free radicals on the collagen molecules. The 1968 paper by Tappel (5) reviews this subject and points out that the animal body, with its many oxygen-labile components, could not exist in its harsh oxidative environment without the presence of biological antioxidants that also serve as free-radical scavengers. Ascorbic acid is intimately involved in this biochemical scheme of natural fat-soluble and water-soluble antioxidants and he states, "Optimum amounts of vitamin C would be important in any attempts to slow the aging processes."

Dr. Alex Comfort, speaking at the Eighth International Conference of Gerontology, also voiced the opinion that antioxidants may retard the aging process (6).

The comprehensive paper by Sokoloff and coworkers (7) at the Southern Bio-Research Institute showed, among other things, that blood-lipid abnormalities increased with advancing age and that ascorbic acid at 2 to 3 grams per day for twelve to thirty months improved this condition in 83 percent of their group of sixty cardiac patients. The 17 percent that showed no effect may have been helped had their hypoascorbemia been fully corrected by the use of more ascorbic acid daily. They also note the need for maintaining the ascorbic acid in the blood and tissues in the antioxidant form by the use of high daily intakes because the oxidized form, dehydroascorbic acid, has undesirable reactions.

There are so many references in the medical literature showing that ascorbic acid requirements are increased in old age and that the elderly suffer from serious depletion, that only a small sampling can be quoted here (8). Yavorsky, Almaden, and King, in 1934, showed that the ascorbic acid content of human tissues decreases with age. The ages varied from one day to seventy-seven years in five groups and the tissues examined included the adrenals, brain, pancreas, liver, spleen, kidney, lung, heart, and thymus. A substantial drop was shown in all cases. Rafsky and Newman, in 1941, examining twenty-five so-called normal individuals, aged sixty to eighty-three, found only two whose ascorbic acid retention behaved normally. Thewlis and Gale concluded, in 1947, that ascorbic acid deficiencies were common in older patients and that:

If there is any chance that a patient may have a cerebral hemorrhage or coronary occlusion, as indicated by high or fluctuating blood pressure, 500 to 1,000 milligrams of ascorbic acid should be given daily, parenterally, for several days.

In a follow-up study published in 1954 of 588 San Mateo County residents over fifty, one of the conclusions of Chope was that low ascorbic acid intake appeared to predispose the sample group to a high mortality. This was confirmed in the 1956 paper by Chope and Breslow. In a comprehensive study on the Nutritional Status of the Aging in California which correlated serum ascorbic acid and intake as reported in 1955 by Morgan and coworkers, good correlation was obtained, but the reported blood serum ascorbic acid values seem too high, indicating that some constant experimental shift to higher values operated during the test. This may be the result of the method they used for the determination of ascorbic acid in the blood serum which includes, besides ascorbic acid, the oxidation products of ascorbic acid itself. This well-planned study should be repeated using an analytical technique which would be utilized to differentiate the presence of reduced ascorbic acid from that of the oxidized form, dehydroascorbic acid, and other decomposition products. This same criticism on the choice of analytical methods applies to many other studies appearing after 1943, when these new analytical techniques were introduced (8).

Other references (9), indicating higher ascorbic acid requirements in the elderly and lower levels found in the body, are Dawson and Bowers, in 1961; and Bowers and Kubik, in 1965; Smolianski, in 1965; Andrews and coworkers, in 1966; O'Sullivan and coworkers, in 1968; Mitra, in 1970; and many more references contained in the bibliographies of these papers.

One paper in this series which should be given special attention is that of Slotkin and Fletcher (10). This paper discussed the stresses of urologic surgery, especially prostatic surgery in patients in their 70s and 80s. Slotkin and Fletcher note that atypical bronchopneumonia is a common and often fatal complication of these operations. These postoperative complications are not truly pneumonic in character, but are the so-called wet chests and foul expectorations due to capillary secretions. They obtained good results, some spectacular, in spite of the pitifully small doses of ascorbic acid employed and concluded: "Irrespective of the blood levels or deficiency of vitamin C, ascorbic acid is a valuable adjunct in tiding these aged patients over their critical postoperative period."

Smolyanskii (11) studied the effect of ascorbic acid on the production of important hormones from the adrenal glands of a group of 144 persons aged 60 to 90 years. He found that both the ascorbic acid blood levels and steroid hormone production were low. A single injection of only 500 milligrams of ascorbic acid increased the urinary excretion of these hormones, indicating a rise in their production by the adrenal gland. Continuing these injections produced further rises in hormone production. It is likely that if these elderly persons had been receiving adequate ascorbic acid over the years, their hormone production would have been maintained at desired youthful levels. The work of Patnaik (11) also indicates a connection between ascorbic acid and aging.

We now have a background of years of highly suggestive research. Yet the crucial tests to determine the actual effects of optimal intakes of ascorbic acid on slowing the aging process have never been started. The genetic rationale for these optimal daily intakes of ascorbic acid for the full correction of the human inborn error of carbohydrate metabolism, hypoascorbemia, is now available (2). The tests would involve simply taking normally healthy age groups and maintaining them for the rest of their lives on ascorbic acid intakes sufficient to fully correct this genetic liver-enzyme disease under conditions of little stress (about 3 to 5 grams of ascorbic acid per day). The health, well-being and mortality of this ascorbic acid group would be compared with similar groups which are solely dependent upon their foodstuffs as their exogenous source of ascorbic acid. The results in a few years may be startling. Time is of the essence in having these tests started. This is the first time that we are in a position to correct this ancient human genetic disease. Let us make the most of it.

19

ALLERGIES, ASTHMA, AND HAY FEVER

An allergy is an abnormal, excessive biochemical response by the body to the introduction of a foreign substance (allergen). It is a bodily defense mechanism which has gotten out of hand. This uncontrolled response manifests itself in many different ways, but they are all basically the same. If the allergen enters through the skin, it may cause rashes or other skin disorders, the so-called contact allergies. If the allergen is a drug or a certain food it may cause digestive upsets and other systemic symptoms of drug or food allergies. Bronchial allergies are termed "asthma." The allergens can also be physical agents, such as heat, cold, or sunlight, which cause unusual, strong reactions in hypersensitive individuals. When the allergen is a skin graft or a transplanted organ, the phenomenon is known as "rejection."

Anaphylactic Shock in Animals

Much work was started in the early 1930s on ascorbic acid's use in anaphylaxis and allergies. Many research reports were published, starting around 1935, and the following is only an incomplete summary of some of the papers. Here, again, a great deal of confusion resulted because many workers reported complete inhibition of the anaphylactic syndrome in experimental animals by ascorbic acid while many others reported no effect. Anaphylaxis or anaphylactic shock is an experimental technique used with test animals because it duplicates the human response in allergies. An animal is given an injection of a foreign substance and, after a suitable incubation period to allow the body's defense mechanism to respond, it is given a second injection of a minute amount of the same foreign substance. The biochemical response of the animal may be so violent that it may quickly die in anaphylactic shock. A review of this early work is found in the 1938 paper by Raffel and Madison, and by Walzer (with ninety references), citing the confusing results of the various workers up to that time (1). Because of the many experimental variables, both controlled and uncontrollable in these tests, many further papers tried to bring some order out of the chaos by involved techniques. Pacheco and coworkers, in 1938, concluded that ascorbic acid has a certain protective action against anaphylactic shock in the guinea pig. Yoshikawa, in 1938, came to a similar conclusion when large doses of ascorbic acid were continuously used, but thought that small doses seemed to increase allergic manifestations (2).

The 1940 paper by Yokoyama (3), of the Kitasato Institute, did much to clear up the importance of the ascorbic acid dosage in preventing death from anaphylactic shock. He took guinea pigs weighing between 200 and 300 grams and sensitized them to horse serum. Three weeks later, he injected them with a minute amount (the minimal lethal dose) of the same horse serum and within a few minutes all the guinea pigs were dead in anaphylactic shock. In other groups of sensitized guinea pigs, he injected ascorbic acid immediately before the same second shocking dose of horse serum. Here are his results as quoted from his paper:

> Thus when 5 to 10 milligrams of ascorbic acid was injected 2 to 3 minutes before the serum injection, shock was not prevented; 20 milligrams delayed death from shock; 30 milligrams prevented shock symptoms and at times prevented shock death, whereas 50 milligrams prevented shock symptoms as well as death from shock in all cases.

If Yokoyama's figures are extrapolated for comparison to the

70-kilogram body weight of an adult human, his ascorbic acid dosages become the following: 2,800 milligrams are completely ineffective; 5,600 milligrams will delay death; 8,400 milligrams will prevent the shock symptoms and sometimes prevent death; 14,000 milligrams will prevent shock symptoms and death and will desensitize the case. This work was confirmed in part by Guirgis, in 1965, and by Dawson and West (3).

The Hungarian workers, Csaba and Toth (4), in 1966, were not able to confirm this work in dogs, but this may have been because they used a shocking dose of horse serum, about 20 to 40 times more than the carefully worked out minimal lethal dose used by Yokoyama (3). Herxheimer (4), in 1965, was also not aware of Yokoyama's effective dosage levels when he reported no anti-anaphylactic effect for ascorbic acid at 10 and 20 milligrams per kilogram body weight.

Hay Fever or Pollinosis

Now let us turn to allergic manifestations in man and look into hay fever, or pollinosis. In 1942 a paper by Holmes and Alexander (5) appeared and gave the results of tests on twenty-five hay fever patients tested consecutively with 100 milligrams of ascorbic acid per day for the first week, 200 milligrams daily for the second week, and finally, 500 milligrams daily for the third week. In most cases, little or no relief was afforded by the 100 milligrams per day level, but when the higher doses were used on the same subjects, they reported a high degree of success, only two of the subjects reporting "no relief." One of the subjects broke out in a rash and quit the test. Holmes extended this work to food allergies and, in 1943, published his results on 27 patients indicating 80 percent success with 500 milligrams of ascorbic acid a day. He notes that while ascorbic acid is nontoxic, he did observe several cases out of a large number where the patients suffered headaches or sore spots around the mouth and, in one instance, diarrhea.

Apparently there is a low percentage in the population of individuals hypersensitive to ascorbic acid who show these reactions to ascorbic acid even though Korbsch (5), in 1938, reported that ascorbic acid in oral doses up to 1 gram a day relieved serum rashes, erythema multiforme (a type of skin rash), and allergic coryza. A possible way of avoiding these reactions may be to build up gradually to the high dosage intakes rather than starting directly with the high levels.

Pelner (6), in 1944, showed that an extremely sensitive ragweed patient could be protected against adverse reactions to pollen-antigen injections by incorporating 100 milligrams of ascorbic acid with the injection. Pelner had also found previously, in 1943, that he could similarly prevent adverse reactions in a series of 51 patients to sulfonamide injections and, in 1942, he prevented the allergic reactions of a rheumatic fever patient to salicylates. Two other papers by Hebald and Engelsher (7) appeared in 1944. Both claimed that ascorbic acid at 500 milligrams per day is not an effective treatment for hay fever. From these contradictory reports, it is evident that 500 milligrams a day is just marginal in hay fever treatment, giving the typical good results with some investigators and outright failures with others. From the lessons learned in Yokoyama's (3) anaphylactic tests on guinea pigs, it is likely that the higher levels of megascorbic therapy would produce more consistent and successful results.

Ruskin, in 1945, concluded as a result of his studies that ascorbic acid plays a valuable role in treating allergies at an optimum dosage of 750 milligrams daily either orally or by injection. In some cases the ascorbic acid therapy alone proved superior to the pollen desensitization used previously. A paper by Friedlander and Feinberg, appearing in 1945, also indicated that 500 milligrams of ascorbic acid daily was insufficient to change the clinical course of hay fever and asthma (8).

Ruskin, 1947, published another paper reporting that sodium ascorbate was more effective than ascorbic acid in refractory cases of allergy and asthma at 1,200 to 1,500 milligrams per day. In 1948, Ruskin published another paper along similar lines and indicated additional successful results. In a study conducted in both Boston and New York on sixty hay fever patients given 1,000 to 2,250 milligrams of ascorbic acid daily along with a few milligrams of vitamin B_1, as reported in 1949, Brown and Ruskin concluded that about 50 percent of their hay fever patients taking the lower dosage and about 75 percent of the patients on the higher doses showed improvement. They stated, "The larger dose may have played a part in producing the apparently greater improvement in the larger percentage of patients." In this test series, one subject reported a laxative effect, two reported flushing and headache, and one reported a rash around the eyes and the scientists stated, "Approximately 5 percent of the patients may suffer mild, although easily controlled, side reactions " (9).

The reader now has a representative review of the clinical research on the use of ascorbic acid in the treatment of hay fever at levels from 100 milligrams to 2,250 milligrams a day. It shows the confusing results at the lower levels of treatment and the greater percentage of success as the dosages were increased. Yet in all these tests the dosages of ascorbic acid used were much below the levels of ascorbic acid indicated by current calculations to be synthesized in the liver of an equivalent-sized mammal under equivalent stress. No one in all these years has been inspired to test dosages of ascorbic acid more closely related to these mammalian levels in spite of the suggestive results of previous clinical tests that the degree of success was dose-related. The protocols of any future clinical tests on hay fever should include the year-round daily intakes of 3 to 5 grams of ascorbic acid, in spaced doses and at higher levels during the particular hay fever season (with and without other antihistamines). The seasonal dosage would be adjusted, depending on the results obtained. If hay fever sufferers were to organize and make enough noise, these tests would be conducted.

Asthma and Bronchospasm

The history of the use of ascorbic acid in the treatment of asthma also dates back to the mid-1930s and is also confusing. It was reviewed in the 1941 paper by Goldsmith (10), who noted the typical pattern of good results of some investigators and of others who failed to confirm these good results. Goldsmith measured the blood ascorbic acid levels of twenty-nine asthmatics and found twenty-two to be below 0.6 mg % (0.7 mg % is considered the minimal normal level) and in two of their patients with hay fever only, ascorbic acid was practically absent from their blood (0.07 and 0.08 mg %). On a regime of 300 milligrams of ascorbic acid daily for 1 week, 200 milligrams daily for the second week, and 50 milligrams daily thereafter, six of seven of their asthmatics were unable to maintain blood levels of 1.0 mg %, which was easily achieved by a healthy control group. They interpreted this as a sign that asthmatics had a greater requirement for ascorbic acid. In some of their patients, they found a relationship between the low blood levels of ascorbic acid and the frequency and severity of asthmatic attacks.

Ten years later, in 1951, the literature was again reviewed by Silbert (10). Of the nineteen papers reviewed, thirteen reported benefit, some to complete remission of symptoms, while 6 reported little or no benefit. Silbert suggested that some of these failures may have been due to inadequate dosages of ascorbic acid.

A series of important papers reporting the work of W. Dawson and coworkers (3,11) on the nature of the antagonism of ascorbate on bronchospasm and on the action of ascorbate on smooth muscle, appeared from 1965 to 1967. They showed that spasmogen-induced broncho-constriction in guinea pigs could be prevented by ascorbic acid. They believed this was due to a direct action of the ascorbate on the bronchial smooth muscle. They also showed that this action is dose-dependent; at low levels it may potentiate the effect of spasmogens, such as histamine, and at higher concentrations it inhibits their spastic effects. This dose-related smooth muscle phenomenon may explain some of the conflicting clinical results of the past four decades.

The protocols for future clinical research using ascorbic acid in asthma should include the megascorbic prophylaxis levels. The dosages would be increased to a point where a therapeutic effect would be obtained. In severe asthmatic attacks, large doses of sodium ascorbate administered intravenously should be tried to relieve the attack. For the safety of this procedure, check the references in Chapter 20 on eye conditions, where doses of 70 grams of sodium ascorbate have been used intravenously without undesirable side effects in the treatment of glaucoma.

Organ Transplants, Skin Grafts, and Rejection

When an organ is transplanted into a body, or even when a piece of skin is grafted onto a damaged surface, there is a very critical initial period of waiting to determine if the organ or the graft "takes." Frequently, there is the possibility that the body may consider the new organ or graft as a foreign substance and begin the allergic, immunological process that is known as rejection. The rejection phenomenon has serious consequences if a vital organ is involved and it may mean a quick death for the individual or, in a skin graft, death to the grafted tissue.

To inhibit the rejection phenomenon, medicine now uses large doses of radiation alone or in combination with the long-term use of various highly toxic, immunosuppressant drugs. Both radiation and these highly toxic drugs are additional biochemical strains on the patient who had undergone complicated surgery. The ascorbic acid levels in these patients, if they were ever measured, would probably be extremely low. These patients, in addition to their other problems, are likely to be suffering from a severe case of uncorrected hypoascorbemia resulting from the stresses of surgery, radiation, and toxic drug administration. Up to the time of this writing, I have been unable to find any reference to the use of large doses of ascorbic acid in the treatment of these patients, either as a nontoxic immunosuppressant or merely to relieve their hypoascorbemia.

Here is a completely unexplored field in organ transplantation and skin grafting which might insure the survival of these patients. In view of the known potential of ascorbic acid in wound healing and of its antiallergic effects when used in the proper large doses, there should be a high priority for tests of massive levels of ascorbic acid to prevent the rejection phenomenon. Animal tests should be started quickly and followed by tests on human transplants.

Protocol for clinical research in this area should include the long-term preoperative daily use of 5 to 10 grams of ascorbic acid, building up to the intravenous use of sodium ascorbate at doses up to possibly 100 or more grams per day intravenously during the postoperative immuno-suppressive phase. If the transplant or grafts "take" under this megascorbic therapy, it may be possible to reduce the ascorbate to a lower holding level.

If this works, it could lead to other valuable pathways, such as the use of high levels of ascorbate in the storage and preservation of organs and the possible use of nonhuman organs to relieve the shortage of human donors.

20

EYE CONDITIONS

Of all the disorders afflicting man, blindness causes the most widespread disability. Aside from the cost in terms of economic loss and the personal expenses of family care and dependency, the annual bill for aid to the blind approaches a billion dollars. It is estimated that a million people in the United States have visual impairment so severe that they cannot read a newspaper. Yet, in spite of significant advances in eye research, the incidence of blindness is increasing. Megascorbic therapy might one day help to reverse this trend.

Structurally, the eye is a spherical camera aimed by exterior muscles. It has a transparent window in the front (cornea) composed of a special protein and a large optic nerve exiting at the rear. The interior is divided into two chambers separated by a flexible lens which focuses the image on a thin, biochemically active membrane (retina) which transforms light energy into nerve impulses. These nerve impulses are gathered into the optic nerve and transmitted to the brain where the color pictures are "seen" and recorded. As would be expected of an organ of such biochemical activity, the eye was early found normally to contain high levels of ascorbic acid and seemed to have the ability to extract it from the blood and to concentrate it for its many vital functions.

The 1962 paper by Heath (1), with forty references to the literature, reviewed the work on ascorbic acid and the eye. He cited twelve separate biochemical processes in which ascorbic acid is involved and speculated on the functions of ascorbic acid in the eye and its possible involvement in diabetic retinopathy, detachment of the retina, and maintenance of the proper consistency of the internal fluids of the eye. It has been known since the early 1930s that ascorbic acid is normally found in the eye at much higher levels than in the blood and in many other tissues. Heath confirmed this by showing that the ascorbic acid levels in different bovine eye tissues were (in milligram percent) the cornea, 30; corneal epithelium, 47 to 94; lens, 34; retina, 22; and were higher than in the skeletal muscle, 2; heart, 4; kidney, 13; and brain 17; but were not as high as in the adrenal gland, 97-160; or the pituitary gland, 126. He states:

> Animals which are capable of synthesizing their own ascorbic acid usually have tissue levels approaching saturation. It would, therefore, seem desirable to insure that the intake of ascorbic acid by man is sufficiently high for tissue saturation. Lower intakes, although not leading to scurvy, may affect some metabolic processes in which ascorbic acid is involved.

Glaucoma

Glaucoma usually appears in middle life and is the second leading cause of blindness in the United States. High pressure within the afflicted eyeball eventually destroys the nerve cells within the retina and progressive loss of vision results. Glaucoma is present in about 2 percent of the population over forty, and 8 to 10 percent over sixty-five. It brings creeping blindness to 3,500 Americans a year.

The prevention of glaucoma is achieved by merely maintaining low intraocular pressure during the lifetime of the individual. The treatment of the disease, once it occurs, is to endeavor to reduce the intraocular pressure to normal levels to prevent further nerve damage. About a million Americans over forty years of age have glaucoma without knowing it. Many cases go undetected for years in spite of the availability of a simple, rapid, and painless tonometer test procedure. Control and prevention of the disease in its early preclinical stages is preferable to waiting for the agony of acute glaucoma to strike.

There was a period of intense research activity from 1964 to 1969 on the use of megascorbic levels of ascorbic acid or sodium ascorbate for reducing the intraocular eye pressure. Linnér (2), in 1964 in Sweden, showed that 0.5 grams of ascorbic acid administered twice daily produced a significant drop in the intraocular pressure of normal eyes. He published another paper, in 1969, in which he showed that 2 grams of ascorbic acid a day, orally, produced the same significant decrease in glaucomatous eyes.

The year 1965 saw the beginning of a four-year period when numerous papers reported on the prompt reduction of the intraocular pressure, with no side effects, by the intravenous injection of 20 percent sodium ascorbate solution at doses of about 70 grams per treatment. Virno and coworkers (3) in Rome published five papers in this period, the group from the University of Rome's Ocular Clinic (4) presented seven papers, one came from Switzerland (5), and one from Finland (5). Even though two papers were published in American journals in 1966 and 1967 by the Italian workers (3), no papers coming from American authors could be found on this exciting line of research.

Such a research silence on the part of American scientists can only be interpreted as an indication that no work has been carried out in the United States in the past six years in this field. Yet, during this same time, numerous government bulletins have appeared describing the urgent need for solving the problem of glaucoma and the daily mail is filled with repeated requests for donations to eye research charities. Where is the money going? What is being done with the available funds?

Research should be started immediately on population groups near forty years of age and older to determine the long-term effect on the inhibition of glaucoma by means of the continued daily intake of about 3 to 5 grams of ascorbic acid. The use of higher dosages, both orally and intravenously, for the therapy of incipient and advanced glaucoma should be included in the research protocols. This will help to determine if a simple and harmless ascorbic acid regimen can be worked out which will prevent blindness in our senior citizens.

Cataracts

A Public Health Service government bulletin (6) starts the discussion of cataracts with:

> Cataracts are the leading cause of blindness in this country. They occur when the chemical composition of the crystalline lens changes, making it opaque rather than transparent. When cataracts form, the only way to restore sight is to remove the afflicted lens. In the majority of cases, cataracts appear to be part of the aging process. Uveitis (inflammation of the eye) and physical and chemical injury are other causes.

Let us discuss these authoritative statements individually:

1. That cataract is now the leading cause of blindness there is no argument—but need it be? The proper long-term use of ascorbic acid may have a profound effect in reducing the incidence of this condition and preventing blindness.

2. Changes in the chemical composition of the lens makes it opaque—correct, no argument. But what is the chemical composition of the lens? It is made from a specially oriented helical protein (7). Dische and Zil (8), in 1951, start their paper, "The most striking chemical change in the lens during the cataractous process is the decrease in sulfhydryl groups." Sulfhydryl groups, like ascorbic acid, are strong, normally occurring reducing agents, and are destroyed by oxidative processes. Possibly, the high levels of ascorbic acid found in the normal eye are there to protect against the loss of these sulfhydryl groups by oxidation. Studies in India (9), from 1963 to 1968, where senile cataract is rampant, occurs at an early age, and matures more quickly, show that cataractous eyes have a much lower content of ascorbic acid than normal eyes. One of these papers (Nema and Srivastava) suggests that the chronically low ascorbic acid content may be responsible for the high incidence of senile cataract.

3. When cataracts form, the only way to restore sight is to remove the afflicted lens—right and wrong. This is the opinion of many present-day ophthalmologists. While some research shows that it is possible to slow down the cataractous process, no work

could be found which would indicate that the proper use of ascorbic acid has been tried to reverse the cataractous process.

4. In the majority of cases, cataracts appear to be part of the aging process—right. But let us do something about this by inhibiting aging (see Chapter 18).

5. Uveitis and physical and chemical injury are other causes—right. All these stresses reduce the ascorbic acid levels in the eye. The 1941 paper of Lyle and McLean of the Royal Air Force on corneal inflammations should not be ignored. They stated:

> Treatment by means of ascorbic acid intravenously is of therapeutic value. The improvement in most cases is almost dramatic. In most cases there is no reason to believe that a general vitamin C deficiency exists. It appears, therefore, that the beneficial results are obtained by flooding the bloodstream with excess of ascorbic acid.

This work was confirmed by Summers in 1946. The profound effects of ascorbic acid on the healing of deep corneal ulcers caused Boyd and Campbell, in 1950, to state and recommend, "We therefore suggest that ascorbic acid, in such massive doses as 1.5 grams daily, has a value in therapy apart from its normal role as a vitamin at accepted levels of intake." The additional work of Campbell and coworkers, in 1950, and Boyd, in 1955, on experimental eye burns, supplies additional confirmation for the need for adequate levels of ascorbic acid in the eye for recovery from heat injury (10).

The answers to this discussion of cataracts seem to be supplied by ascorbic acid. Are they not sufficiently suggestive to warrant further research and investigation?

The literature cited in this discussion of cataracts is but a small fraction of the total which has been published on ascorbic acid and the eye since the early 1930s. To thoroughly review this voluminous work is beyond the scope of a short monograph. We have to omit the work done on experimental diabetic cataracts, naphthalene cataracts, and dinitrophenol cataracts. But before closing this chapter, let us consider only four of the papers on senile cataract.

As long ago as 1939, Muhlmann and coworkers (11), in the Argentine, obtained 90 percent good results in sixty patients with 113 incipient senile cataracts by 2 series of daily injections, for ten days each, of 50 to 100 milligrams of ascorbic acid. He concluded that the treatment had no contraindications, should be tried in all incipient cases, and is more effective the earlier it is used.

In another 1939 paper, "Vitamin C and the Aging Eye," Bouton (11) of Detroit found "ascorbic acid deficiency can be held partly responsible for impairment of vision associated with senescence of the human eye and that the administration of ascorbic acid by mouth can counteract this process." He gave 350 milligrams of ascorbic acid a day for four to eight weeks and obtained improvement in vision in 60 percent of the treated group; marked improvement usually set in within the first two weeks of treatment. He believed that cataracts already formed were not affected and the benefits obtained were due to clearing of the other optic media and to some degree to a beneficial effect on the retinal vessels and the head of the optic nerve. While 350 milligrams of ascorbic acid a day was considered a huge dose in 1939, the administration of multigram daily levels would have obtained even better results.

Atkinson, an ophthalmologist of more than thirty years' experience, published, in 1952, a scholarly paper on the senile cataract (11). He stated, ". . . in a larger percentage of cases than most surgeons have realized, cataract is a preventable disease." In 1952 he had over 450 cases of incipient cataract under his treatment which included, among other dietary suggestions, the administration of about 1 gram of ascorbic acid a day. He noted that untreated incipient cataracts matured in four years or less, some taking only one year. Of his over 450 patients under prophylaxis, only a limited number matured and went on to surgery, whereas formerly nearly all had to submit to surgery. He states that in a number of his patients the cataracts have remained incipient over a period of eleven years.

The promising leads relating to ascorbic acid cited above, have not been picked up or been the subject of intensive research in an effort to help prevent this annual plague of blindness. Why? A search of the government bulletin (6) entitled, "Research Profile— Summary of Progress in Eye Disorders," discussed before, fails to reveal a single mention of ascorbic acid in its 16 pages. This indicates that no research on the use of ascorbic acid for the prevention of blindness is being conducted at the National Institutes of Health or the National Institute of Neurological Diseases and Blindness. The same situation probably exists in the research facilities of the many publicly supported charitable foundations for the blind.

Most of the investigators using ascorbic acid in the treatment of eye pathology employed it orally or by injection. It is also possible to use it as a solution of sodium ascorbate applied topically. This is especially effective when the topical application is done iontophoretically. This method uses a harmless mild electric current to force the ascorbate into the eye tissues. As pointed out by Erlanger (12), in 1954, after many years of research, iontophoresis is another neglected principle of therapy which should find much wider use in the treatment of eye diseases. Topical megascorbic therapy and iontophoresis should be a most valuable combination.

Retinal Detachment

Another area for eye research is in retinal detachments. A 1964 paper by Weber and Wilson (12) showed that the ascorbic acid levels in the subretinal fluid decreased with the length of time of the retinal detachments. Possibly, individuals on high levels of ascorbic acid would have less chance of suffering retinal detachment. The research on this condition could be combined with the above suggested tests on glaucoma and cataracts to determine whether the prophylactic daily dosage of 3 to 5 grams of ascorbic acid would also reduce the incidence of retinal detachments.

21

ULCERS

Peptic ulcers may be the butt of many jokes, but as any ulcer sufferer can testify, having one is not funny. Ulcers are a painful, chronic disease affecting about 14 million Americans during their productive years. Every day some 4,000 individuals develop an ulcer and each year about 10,000 people die of complications from peptic ulcer. The drain on the economy is estimated to be 500 million dollars in lost man-hours and cost of medical treatment. A simple, inexpensive, successful preventive and therapeutic regime is needed.

Our stomach is the second stop in the processing of food for digestion and absorption. It is a tough, strong, muscular, spheroidal-shaped bag with an opening at the top (inlet) and at the side (outlet). Each opening is surrounded by a circular muscle, the sphincter, controlled by nerve impulses for opening and closing. The top opening is connected to the esophagus, which carries the food from the mouth; the side opening is connected to the duodenum, the first section of the intestines. The lining of the stomach secretes strong hydrochloric acid and a powerful enzyme, pepsin, which dissolves and digests proteins.

The stomach contents are normally highly irritating, corrosive, and erosive. This can be seen when the stomach contents sometimes back up into the esophagus producing the distressing sensations of "heartburn" and in the sour, irritating taste of vomit. Since the stomach walls are themselves made of protein, they must in some way be protected against the corrosive action of their own secretions. Sometimes this equilibrium is disrupted and open sores and lesions in the lining result. If they are in the stomach, they are called gastric ulcers; if in the adjacent intestine, duodenal ulcers. In the United States, duodenal ulcers are about eight times more common than gastric ulcers.

The secretion of hydrochloric acid and the enzyme, pepsin, is also under nervous control. The stimulation of these nerves is caused by food entering the mouth or even by the thought of food, so that the stomach will be ready for processing the food when it reaches there. In nervous people, smokers, excessive drinkers, or individuals under stress, this nervous stimulation does not turn off at the proper sequence or turns on when there is no food in the stomach. When no food is present to take the full brunt of the corrosive chemical attack of the stomach juices, gastric distress is felt and, if long continued, actual attack of the lining may result.

Animal experiments have been conducted since the early 1930s on ascorbic acid and its relation to gastric and duodenal ulcers. In 1933, Smith and McConkey (1), working in a New York State tuberculosis hospital, performed autopsies on 1,000 guinea pigs that had been fed a normal diet and failed to find a single spontaneous stomach ulcer. Of seventy-five guinea pigs fed a diet deficient in ascorbic acid, twenty, or approximately twenty-six percent, developed ulcers. In eighty guinea pigs fed the same deficient diet but supplemented with added ascorbic acid, only one developed ulcers. In other experiments, they found that diets deficient in vitamins A, B, and D did not produce ulcers if the ascorbic acid supply was adequate. Mechanical injury to the duodenum lining of guinea pigs fed an adequate diet was followed by rapid and complete healing, while similar injury to guinea pigs on an ascorbic acid-deficient diet resulted in the formation of duodenal ulcers. They also gave a small group of their tuberculous patients with chronic duodenal ulcers tomato juice supplements (their only source of ascorbic acid in those early days) with favorable responses. They also advised adding tomato juice or orange juice to the scurvy-producing Sippy or Lenhartz diets used for ulcer treatment. Hanke (1), in Germany in 1937, confirmed this work.

There is an extensive medical literature on clinical tests going as far back as 1934 correlating deficiency of ascorbic acid with high incidence of gastric and duodenal ulcers, bleeding ulcers, and poor healing after surgery. Many of the papers point out that the ulcer patient should receive adequate amounts of ascorbic acid.

Over the years, the author has collected over fifty medical research papers on this subject with no claim that this represents all the papers which have been published. Complete reference to all these papers is obviously beyond the scope and space of this book. Instead, a limited illustrative selection of twelve papers is included in the bibliography covering the period from 1936 to 1968 (2). The earliest papers show that ulcer patients have higher requirements for ascorbic acid than normal subjects. The patients have low, inadequate intakes of ascorbic acid and are in a state of subclinical scurvy and there is poor healing of the ulcers and the wounds after surgery. The papers recommend that ulcer patients receive plenty of ascorbic acid. The following are quotes from a few of these early papers:

It is important for the clinician to make sure that patients with peptic ulcers are receiving an adequate amount of vitamin C ... The severest degrees of vitamin C deficiency were found in the patients with haematemesis (vomiting of blood). It is suggested that large doses of vitamin C should be given to all subjects of peptic ulceration and haematemesis in order to saturate them as rapidly as possible (2).

The results and suggestions contained in these early references have been repeated in the later papers and have continued up to the present time.

In 1968, Russell and coworkers (2) compared a series of sixty hospitalized patients with gastrointestinal hemorrhage—2 with peptic ulcer—with a group having uncomplicated peptic ulcer and with healthy controls. They found significantly lower ascorbic acid levels in the bleeding group than in the uncomplicated peptic ulcer group, which was much lower than the healthy controls. The differences were more striking with advancing age over forty-five. They stated that only six of the bleeders had any clinical evidence of scurvy but that the rest suffered from a subclinical form of the disease. They believed this subclinical scorbutic state prevented healing of the bleeding ulcers and maintained hemorrhage in the gastric erosions precipitated by other factors such as aspirin or alcohol.

Certain drugs, such as aspirin, cortisone, and other anti-inflammatory agents, and cinchophen, are known to provoke ulcers and gastric hemorrhage. This is especially the case when a deficiency of ascorbic acid is present. In animal experiments, the administration of ascorbic acid along with the toxic drug reduced the incidence of peptic ulcer and gastric hemorrhage to such an extent that it prompted one author (Aron) to suggest, "Therefore it would seem judicious in human therapeutics to include ascorbic acid in every prescription for an anti-inflammatory drug" (3).

In any surgery, the importance of ascorbic acid has long been known (see Chapter 27). Patients undergoing surgery for ulcers are no exception. In a 1947 paper, Zerbini (4) discusses two surgical cases of patients with ascorbic acid deficiency. One patient exhibited severe surgical shock during the operation and the other patient showed no evidence of healing of the surgical wounds when the stitches were removed on the seventh postoperative day. This latter patient had been given a daily injection of 200 milligrams of ascorbic acid, but obviously this low, vitaminlike dosage was insufficient to supply the patient's high demands and as a result the wounds did not heal.

Williamson, in 1967, again confirmed the low ascorbic acid levels in patients subjected to gastric surgery and said that in these patients, "the administration of ascorbic acid would seem obligatory." Cohen, in the same year, stated that all patients with gastrointestinal disorders should be suspected of having subclinical scurvy. He also pointed out that this concept was proposed by Lazarus in 1937 but was "not yet generally acknowledged." This was over three decades ago—the medical mills certainly grind slowly. Three other papers and a review added further confirmation to the pathogenetic role played by low levels of ascorbic acid in gastrointestinal disorders. In the paper by Cohen and Duncan they state:

> [Patients should] be given routine ascorbic acid supplements before surgery and during the phase of early wound healing. . . .

There are no known hazards of ascorbic acid therapy, and overdosage is therefore of no practical importance (4).

In a thirteen-page government bulletin (5) entitled "Peptic Ulcer," prepared by The National Institute of Arthritis and Metabolic Diseases of the National Institutes of Health, there is not a single mention of ascorbic acid in the entire booklet. Nothing is said of its possible role in ulcer formation or in the ulcer treatment, in spite of the worldwide background of nearly four decades of research, some of which has been cited above. This is a bulletin sold to the general public for its information on the causes and treatments of this disease. "The Medical Letter," which is a semimonthly publication for doctors and is designed to convey authoritative recommendations for current medical treatments, devoted a large part of its December 26, 1969, issue to a discussion of the "Medical Treatment of Peptic Ulcer " (5). Here again no mention is made of ascorbic acid in the two and a half pages of discussion. It seems rather fantastic that, in both these publications, all of the suggestive work reported in the medical literature on ascorbic acid in ulcer therapy, can be so blatantly ignored. It also indicates that the use of ascorbic acid in ulcer therapy is not widely practiced and that ulcer patients are generally denied the possible benefits indicated in the above review of medical literature.

The following clinical research proposal is made in the hope that it will be picked up and tested by the government health agencies, by the publicly endowed health foundations with clinical testing facilities, or by doctors in the gastrointestinal field. The proposed rationale for the use of sodium ascorbate instead of ascorbic acid in ulcer prevention and therapy at megascorbic levels combines the antacid and buffering capacity of sodium ascorbate with its wound healing and antihemorrhagic effects. The research protocol would include the use of 0.5 to 1 teaspoonful (1.5 to 4 grams) of sodium ascorbate, dissolved in a glass of milk, taken before meals and at bedtime. For gastric distress at other times, 0.5 teaspoon of sodium ascorbate, dissolved in about 2 ounces of water, will usually provide immediate relief. This simple regime was very successful in several ulcer volunteers who were thus able to avoid surgery. The use of sodium ascorbate should be subjected to large-scale clinical testing to determine its value as a new approach to peptic ulcer prevention and therapy.

22

KIDNEYS AND BLADDER

It has been estimated that about 100,000 deaths occur each year in this country as a result of various diseases of the kidneys or their complications. Kidney and related diseases are the main cause of work loss among American women. About 3.5 million Americans have unrecognized and undiagnosed infections of the kidneys and urinary tract. Painful symptoms will prompt some to seek medical advice but others, a significant number, will have no warning until the damage has reached an advanced stage. An effective prophylactic regime is, therefore, urgently needed.

The kidneys are complex biochemical organs serving mainly to regulate and maintain our internal environment. They do this by varying the volume of the urine and the secretion into it of various bodily waste products which would otherwise pollute our system. The two, purplish-brown, bean-shaped, depolluting kidneys are located in the small of the back and are equipped with a large blood supply. The renal artery brings the polluted blood to the kidney and the renal vein carries away the purified blood. The urine, produced by a complex filtration system in the kidney, is collected into a duct called the ureter, which carries the fluid to the bladder for storage. Another tube, called the urethra, carries the urine to the outside for disposal. Because of an evolutionary anatomical compromise of Nature, the final urinary structures are tied in with the reproductive organs, which complicates an already complex system. The entire structure from the kidneys to the exit tubes is called the genito-urinary tract.

The megascorbic treatment rationale for many urological, renal, or genito-urinary diseases would comprise the following steps and the body's resulting physiological responses. Large doses of ascorbic acid are administered, preferably orally and in solution, at frequent intervals. The doses will be of the order of 2 grams about every two hours. It is conveniently given by dissolving about a 0.5 teaspoonful of ascorbic acid in about four ounces of fruit or tomato juice or in about two ounces of water sweetened to taste with sugar or artificial sweetener. The ascorbic acid could also be given parenterally if the physician desires.

The ascorbic acid will be rapidly absorbed and will enter the bloodstream causing a rise in the ascorbic acid blood levels to above the kidney threshold. The kidneys start pulling it out of the blood and excreting it into the urine. This removal by the kidneys continues and before the blood is exhausted another large dose of administered ascorbic acid maintains the excretory function at a high rate. The ascorbic acid level in the urine builds up to a concentration where it can exert bacteriostatic, bactericidal, and virucidal effects. Phagocytes in adjacent tissues would be stimulated to efficiently digest any bacteria.

Here, then, we have a situation where the complete genito-urinary tract from the renal tubules to the urethra would be continuously bathed in a fluid that is bactericidal and virucidal, and has detoxicating and wound-healing properties. Infections of the urinary tract should be more easily controlled through the use of this regimen. If antibiotics or other medicaments are employed, the ascorbic acid should aid and potentiate their effects. There do not seem to be any predictable contraindications to its use as an adjuvant treatment. The continued presence of high levels of ascorbic acid in the urine in contact with all these tissues should prevent any incipient infections from developing.

For urological surgery a suggested program could include

maintaining the patient on a preoperative schedule of about half the suggested dosage level for a few days to a week before surgery. During and after surgery the dosage schedule should be maintained and continued until healing is complete. The patient may then be put on a maintenance dose of about 5 grams per day. All these doses are only suggested starting points and may be varied as experience dictates.

A simple prophylactic regime to prevent the incidence and recurrence of kidney diseases could be based on the maintenance of high levels of ascorbic acid in the urine. This could be accomplished by the long-term use of ascorbic acid, about 3 to 5 grams a day in three to five spaced doses. Large-scale clinical testing of this simple regimen would provide the statistics to determine its usefulness.

Bladder Tumors

In 1969, Schlegel, Pipkin, and coworkers (1), at Tulane University School of Medicine, summarized the results of their research on bladder tumor formation. They demonstrated that the oral administration of large quantities of ascorbic acid, sufficient to produce a significant rise in the ascorbic acid content of the urine, will prevent the development of bladder cancer. They suggest the daily intake of 1.5 grams of ascorbic acid in three spaced doses for "individuals who, due to age, cigarette smoking, or other factors, may be prone to bladder tumor formation."

Renal Failure

Another area in which ascorbic acid may be useful and has been practically unexplored is in renal failure. When renal failure occurs, the kidneys malfunction and various chemical imbalances are produced in the blood which can be fatal. Heroic measures may be necessary to save the patient. One of the measures involves connecting the patient's blood system to an artificial kidney machine, if one is available, to take over the functions of the damaged kidney. This is called "hemodialysis." The machine purifies the polluted blood and returns the purified blood to the patient. Until the kidney becomes normal again, the patient must make repeated trips to the machine in order to remain alive, which is a rather expensive and tedious procedure.

In 1968 and 1970, it was shown that, when patients are connected to the kidney machines, the hemodialysis not only removes the undesirable products from the blood but also removes a substantial proportion of the patient's already low stores of ascorbic acid (2). Replacement of his ascorbic acid is needed and page 1345 of the 1970 paper states:

Since ascorbic acid lost from the plasma during dialysis is not adequately replaced by dietary consumption of vitamin C, patients undergoing maintenance hemodialysis should receive ascorbic acid supplementation as an important part of their therapeutic regimen.

Further clinical studies should be conducted on this renal failure to determine the effect of continued daily megascorbic dosages, both orally and intravenously, on the detoxifying effects of ascorbic acid in relieving the build-up of toxic materials in the blood. If ascorbic acid can control this toxic burden, it might mean fewer trips to the scarce kidney machines with consequently less stress on the patient and his pocketbook.

Neglected but highly significant observations on rabbits with both kidneys removed, published in 1950 by Mason, Casten, and Lindsay (2), supply additional incentive for more research on the possible usefulness of ascorbic acid in kidney failure. Rabbits with both kidneys surgically removed uniformly die in three to four days. If, however, these animals without kidneys are injected with a mixture of ascorbic acid and p-aminobenzoic acid, the scientists state:

The duration of survival was strikingly increased, ranging from five and a half to eight and a half days. Even more striking was the improved condition of the animals during most of the period of survival. They were alert, active, and in most respects behaved like normal rabbits until a few hours prior to death.

In kidney transplantation the possibility of using megascorbic levels of ascorbic acid has never been adequately explored. The maintenance of these high levels may reduce the occurrence of rejection reactions and certainly would help insure survival of the patient by counteracting the effects of surgical shock, promoting kidney function during recovery, and aiding in wound healing. The kidney research on ascorbic acid should be oriented toward the prevention of kidney damage by continued use of ascorbic acid

and, if kidney damage is already present, to determine if biochemical repair can be effected. In this way, the expensive trauma of
hemodialysis and transplantation could possibly be avoided. There
are many publicly supported foundations and government agencies
which could undertake this work.

Stone Formation

A criticism that has been leveled against supplying to humans
the daily amounts of ascorbic acid which are normally produced in
other mammals is that its acidifying effect on the urine might
increase the incidence of stone formation. The formation of stones
in the urinary tract is a very complex subject and intensive and
large-scale research should be conducted to resolve this important
question.

Abundant archaeological evidence indicates that stone formation
is among the oldest afflictions of man. It is common today in
all parts of the world and in some areas of the world the incidence
is so high that they are known as "stone belts." In the 1964 paper,
containing a bibliography of 104 references, Gershoff (3) states,
"Urinary calculi vary so much in form, occurrence, and composition that it is unlikely that a single mechanism is responsible for
their production." The composition depends on whether it is a
kidney stone or a bladder stone and in what part of the world the
individual lives. About 1 percent of the 280,000 surgical cases
admitted to the London Hospital from 1906 to 1935 were for
stones of the urinary tract. In 25,000 autopsies at the University of
Minnesota hospitals, the incidence of kidney stones was 1.12 percent. The incidence varies considerably in different parts of the
world with a high percentage of bladder stones in children one to
ten years old in Thailand, India, Syria, China, and Turkey. In an
analysis of 1,000 urinary stones from the United States, 52 percent
contained phosphates, 33 percent were calcium oxalate, 6 percent
were urate stones, and 3 percent cystine. Because of the wide
variation in composition, the acidifying effect of ascorbic acid in
the urine may inhibit stone formation of certain types, especially
those containing phosphates, which comprise a large fraction of
those found in American urinary stones. McCormick (4), in 1947,
surveyed the worldwide incidence of stone formation and his own
clinical experience and experimentation, and he concluded that

stone formation (urinary, salivary, biliary, and so on) was due to a deficiency of ascorbic acid. He pointed out that administration of ascorbic acid had profound effects on urinary sedimentation and crystallization. He states: "As soon as corrective administration of the vitamin effects a normal ascorbic acid level, the crystalline and organic sediment disappears like magic from the urine. I have found that this change can usually be brought about in a matter of hours by large doses of the vitamin—500 to 2,000 milligrams—oral or parenteral. Subsequent maintenance doses of 100 to 300 milligrams, daily, are usually sufficient to keep the urine free from these deposits. It would thus appear that deficiency of vitamin C, which is the predominating dietary defect in the various 'stone areas,' may provide the predominating factor in urinary lithogenesis [stone formation]."

Most people do not drink enough water and this is a neglected and little explored factor in stone formation. It is common knowledge that the tendency for salts to crystallize out of solution is greater the more concentrated the solution is. In people whose water intake is low, the urine is much more concentrated. In the "stone belts" of the world, water is scarce and of poor quality, and the climate is hot, so most of the population is in a chronic state of water deprivation. In Israel, where there is a high incidence of urinary stone formation, Frank and coworkers (5) were able to reduce the incidence of stone formation by merely educating the settlers to drink more water. They stated, "Preliminary results, summarizing a 3-year period of study, suggest that education is capable of raising urine output and preventing urolithiasis (urinary stone formation) in a hot, dry climate." It is likely that copious daily intakes of good soft drinking water along with the high ascorbic acid intakes would tend to correct any individual tendency to stone formation. The author, who has been ingesting high levels of ascorbic acid for over three decades and has not been troubled with stone formation, also tries to drink at least a quart of water a day in addition to other fluids. Large-scale clinical studies should be started to obtain further data because there are probably millions of Americans taking high levels of ascorbic acid on their own volition.

Several minor studies on urinary oxalate excretion have already been made because oxalate formation is a possible result of ascorbic acid breakdown in the body and calcium oxalate is a constituent of many human stones. In a test on 51 male subjects reported in 1954 by Lamden and coworkers (6), results showed that the daily ingestion of up to 4 grams of ascorbic acid a day produced no significant increase in oxalate excretion. Eight grams a day produced an average increase of 45 milligrams a day and 9 grams increased average oxalate excretion by 68 milligrams a day. The range of urinary oxalate excretion of the subjects *before* taking the ascorbic acid was 10 to 64 milligrams per day. The normal individual variations among their subjects, of 54 milligrams a day, was thus greater than the average increase in excretion found for the 8-gram ascorbic acid test intake. Two papers from Japan in 1966 and one from Egypt (6), in 1970, reported similar additional results. Takenouchi and coworkers reported that 3 grams of ascorbic acid produced no marked increases in oxalate excretion in three subjects, while 9 grams a day increased it to 20 to 30 milligrams a day. The variation in oxalate excretion of their three subjects *before* taking the ascorbic acid (11 to 64 milligrams per day) was even greater than the increase found for the 9-gram intake. Takaguchi and coworkers gave their three groups of ten subjects 1 and 2 grams of ascorbic acid daily for 90 to 180 days. They found no significant increase in urinary oxalate excretion. The normal oxalate excretion of their subjects on the same standardized diet before taking the ascorbic acid varied from a low of 11 milligrams to a high of 55 milligrams. El-Dakhakhny and El-Sayed fed 4 grams of ascorbic acid to 8 subjects on the same diet whose urinary oxalate excretion before the ascorbic acid varied from 17 to 132 milligrams per day. In one subject there was no change, in two subjects there was a decrease of 32 to 56 milligrams, while in the other five, increases of 10 to 18 milligrams a day were reported. Evidently there are many other factors beside ascorbic acid that determine urinary oxalate.

While cystine stones are relatively rare, the megascorbic approach to their control has never been considered before. Cystine is the insoluble, oxidized form of the acid-soluble, sulfur amino acid cysteine. The soluble form (cysteine) is a strong reducing agent, like ascorbic acid, and both cysteine and ascorbic acid are members of normal biological oxidation-reduction systems. They both interact and protect each other from the bad effects of oxidation. Maintenance of high levels of the highly reducing ascorbic acid in the urinary system of cystinurics (those people prone to cystine stones) may make it possible to maintain their abnormally high cysteine levels in the reduced soluble form and thus avoid conversion to the insoluble cystine, with subsequent crystallization and stone formation. In this way, the excess cysteine could be disposed of in a reduced soluble form in the ascorbic acid-acidified urine. This is similar to the rationale proposed by Schlegel, Pipkin and coworkers (1) who utilized the antioxidant effect of ascorbic acid in the prevention of bladder cancer. This rationale for cystine stone prevention is an entirely new area of clinical research resulting from these megascorbic concepts.

23

DIABETES AND HYPOGLYCEMIA

Diabetes and its opposite counterpart, hypoglycemia, are diseases caused by disturbances in the delicate balance of the sugar chemistry of the body. The sugar, glucose, is a normal blood constituent and is used by the body as a source of energy. To utilize this energy the body requires insulin and some 20 enzymatic chemical reactions.

For the normal functioning of the human body, the concentration of glucose in the blood must be maintained within narrow limits (the normal range is 80 to 120 mg %). The biochemical traffic policeman that controls the level of glucose in the blood is insulin. Insulin is produced in a part of the pancreas called the Islets of Langerhans, from where it enters the bloodstream.

Since the amount of glucose in the blood may vary, such as after eating, the insulin must be doled out by the pancreas in just the right amounts. Too little insulin circulating in the blood permits the glucose levels to rise (hyperglycemia) and brings on the diabetic state. When the blood level of glucose rises above the height of the kidney dam of 170 mg % (kidney threshold) it spills over into the urine and positive urinary sugar tests result. Too much insulin in the blood is equally bad because it produces the condition of hypoglycemia (low blood sugar) and there are probably as many people suffering from this serious condition as from diabetes.

In the treatment of diabetes, insulin is injected because, if given orally, it is destroyed by the digestive enzymes. The dosage of insulin requires careful control because if it is too much, low blood sugar, or "insulin shock," will result. A test used to determine whether pancreatic secretion of insulin is normal or not is the so-called glucose-tolerance test. A large amount of glucose sugar is fed the fasting patient. The blood glucose values are determined before and at hourly intervals after ingesting the sugar. From the result obtained it is possible to distinguish normality, diabetes (too little insulin), and hypoglycemia (too much insulin). If the body has an excess of sugar beyond its immediate needs, it is converted to the insoluble carbohydrate, glycogen, which is deposited in the liver for storage. Thus a sugar reserve is available and, in times of need, glycogen can be converted back into the soluble sugar, glucose.

An estimated 4 million Americans have diabetes and about ½ of these are undiagnosed. Heredity is important because, in about 50 percent of the cases, there is a familial history of diabetes. It has also been estimated that about 22 percent of the United States population carries the recessive gene for this disease. Diabetes ranks eighth as a cause of death in the United States and it is the third leading cause of blindness. The importance of maintaining the delicate biochemical balance of insulin, therefore, cannot be underrated. The use of insulin for the treatment of diabetes began in the 1920s and the Canadians, Frederick Banting and John Macleod, received the 1923 Nobel Prize in Biochemistry for its discovery.

Not long after the discovery of ascorbic acid in the early 1930s, tests on guinea pigs indicated that ascorbic acid had a profound influence on the body's sugar utilization. In 1934, C. G. King and coworkers (1), at the University of Pittsburgh, showed that guinea pigs maintained on low levels of ascorbic acid developed degeneration of the Islets of Langerhans. Guinea pigs depleted of ascorbic acid showed a low glucose tolerance which was rapidly regained on feeding them ascorbic acid. In 1935 and 1937, they also demonstrated that injection of sublethal doses of diphtheria toxin (increased stress) further diminished their tolerance to sugar in proportion to the length of their ascorbic acid deprivation.

These results were confirmed and extended in a comprehensive series of papers from India by Banerjee (2), starting in 1943. He not only confirmed that guinea pigs with scurvy showed poor sugar tolerance, but indicated that the insulin content of the pancreas of scorbutic guinea pigs is reduced to about ⅛ that of normal guinea pigs. He observed gross changes in the microscopic appearance of sections of the pancreas from scorbutic guinea pigs. The appearance returned to normal when the guinea pigs were given ascorbic acid. He also reported that the normal conversion of excess sugar into glycogen reserves for liver storage is also impaired in scurvy. In 1947, using improved laboratory techniques, he confirmed his earlier results and revised his estimate of the insulin content of the pancreas of scorbutic guinea pigs to one-quarter that of normal. He also states in this paper:

> The disturbed carbohydrate metabolism as seen in scurvy is due to a deficiency of insulin secretion and a chronic deficiency of this vitamin may be one of the etiological factors (causes) of diabetes mellitus in human subjects.

In 1958, he published the results of additional studies which confirmed his earlier work. His 1964 paper contained the very suggestive results of the work on the intestinal transport of glucose. It was found that the intestinal absorption of sugar was about doubled when the animals were deprived of ascorbic acid and returned to normal when they received ascorbic acid. If this observation is applicable to humans, it would mean that the intestines of diabetics, who may exist on chronic, low levels of ascorbic acid, would permit much more rapid absorption of sugar after eating. The blood sugar levels would rise to higher levels faster and put abnormal stress on the already strained insulin production in their pancreas.

Other workers have reached similar results. In fact, there have been so many papers published that a complete review is impossible in a single chapter. We will only discuss some very suggestive results on which further research should be expended. Altenburger, in 1936, showed that guinea pigs deprived of ascorbic acid were unable to convert glucose to glycogen for storage in their livers, but this condition was promptly relieved when ascorbic acid was administered. A dose of insulin that produced a pronounced decline in blood sugar in normal monkeys had little effect on monkeys deprived of ascorbic acid (Stewart and coworkers, 1952).

The intimate relationship between insulin and ascorbic acid has been noted numerous times. When insulin is injected, there is a fall in the ascorbic acid levels in the blood serum of man, dogs, and rats, as shown by Ralli and Sherry in 1940 and 1948. Haid, in 1941, also noted this drop, not only after insulin injection but in patients in insulin shock. Previously, in 1939, Wille reported that ascorbic acid is helpful to schizophrenics receiving insulin shock treatments. She also produced evidence that ascorbic acid acts to raise the blood sugar levels in hypoglycemic attacks and said that prolonged administration of ascorbic acid will prevent these low blood sugar attacks (3).

Ascorbic acid potentiates the action of insulin and, therefore, makes it possible to derive the same effect with much less insulin. This was observed in 1939 by Bartelheimer and was accidently confirmed by Rogoff and coworkers in 1944 (4). Rogoff and his coworkers noted greater sensitivity in two diabetic children to their usual dose of insulin in the diabetic ward of their Pittsburgh hospital. On checking, they found that the children had also been given ascorbic acid and they believed this fact was responsible for the excessive insulin effect. In reviewing the literature, they cite a paper by Dienst, Diemer, and Scheer which reported that the ascorbic acid used in their tests on diabetics was equivalent to the effect of twenty units of insulin. They also mention the work of Pfleger and Scholl (4) who, in 1937, noted that ascorbic acid so improved the action of insulin that a diabetic could control his sugar tolerance with a lower level of insulin. Such conclusions should have initiated large-scale intensive research to determine how much ascorbic acid is needed to minimize the disagreeable insulin injections and still maintain controlled sugar metabolism and, incidently, save diabetics millions of dollars. The combination of ascorbic acid with the oral medications may also be helpful in avoiding some of the undesirable vascular side effects of diabetic treatment (5).

Tests were started in the early 1930s to determine if the administration of ascorbic acid would reduce the blood sugar levels of diabetics and this resulted in a large volume of medical literature. As in the treatment of other diseases, with the short-term use of ascorbic acid, the more papers that appeared, the more confusion resulted. Some clinicians reported good results in controlling diabetes and others stated that there was no effect. The pros and cons are too numerous to be reviewed here. It was pointed out, in 1935, that the doses used may have been insufficient (6). Whether or not this was true is unimportant; the entire approach to this research work may have been misdirected. The tests were aimed at the short-term application of ascorbic acid to see whether diabetes, caused by an already damaged pancreas, could be controlled. A better approach would have been in the area of prevention: the long-term administration of ascorbic acid to prevent pancreatic damage and the subsequent occurrence of diabetes. Such a plan is explained in the following paragraphs.

There is an assemblage of facts, scattered in the medical literature like pieces of a jigsaw puzzle, which have lain dormant for decades. But when put together, they form the picture for research to possibly prevent the millions of cases of diabetes which develop later in life, especially in individuals who carry the recessive gene for this trait. The pattern of the projected research would be to correct one genetic disease, hypoascorbemia, in order to help prevent the other, diabetes. Here are the facts.

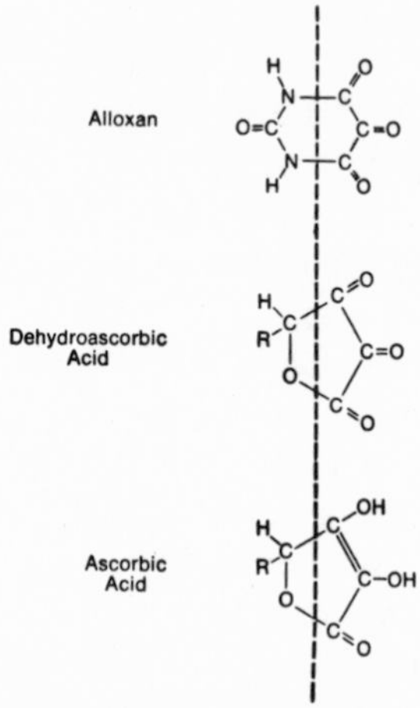

Figure 6   Similarity of Molecular Structure of Alloxan and Dehydroascorbic Acid, Especially to Right of Dashed Center Line

1. There is a substance called alloxan which, when injected into laboratory animals, produces diabetes. This has long been known and was used as far back as 1943 as a convenient and rapid means for inducing diabetes in laboratory animals for testing purposes.

2. When ascorbic acid is oxidized, it forms dehydroascorbic acid, a compound similar in structure to alloxan. The structures of ascorbic acid, dehydroascorbic acid and alloxan are shown in Figure 6. One doesn't have to be a chemist to see the similarity between dehy-

droascorbic acid and alloxan structures to the right of the midline drawn through the molecule and the dissimilarity of ascorbic acid. The chemical properties of alloxan and dehydroascorbic acid are also strikingly similar, as noted by Patterson in 1950.

3. Like alloxan, the injection of dehydroascorbic acid into rats produces diabetes as was shown by Patterson in 1949 and also produces diabetic cataracts as he showed in 1951. That injection of ascorbic acid does not produce diabetes was shown by Levey and Suter in 1946.

4. Banerjee reported in 1952 that he found no dehydroascorbic acid in the tissues, including the pancreas, of normal guinea pigs but stated, "It was present in considerable amounts in the tissues of scorbutic guinea pigs" (7).

5. The mammalian genetic disease, hypoascorbemia, prevents us from making the mammalian liver metabolite, ascorbic acid. The full correction of this genetic disease provides the rationale for the intake of much higher levels of ascorbic acid (8).

The genetically potential diabetics are those who may develop the diabetic state later in life. During their early years, they have an apparent normal production and secretion of insulin from their pancreas. As a group, they are likely to be more sensitive to factors which may affect the delicate physiological balance which controls insulin production. This is indeed a delicate equilibrium. With too little insulin, diabetes is the result; too much insulin produces the equally serious disease, hypoglycemia. These genetically sensitive individuals have probably existed all of their lifetime on suboptimal levels of ascorbic acid. Even the best diet could not supply their individual requirements. Finally, chronic ascorbic acid deprivation and depletion pushes them over the brink into a state of abnormal insulin production. This chronic exposure of their pancreas to the consequent high ratios of dehydroascorbic acid may slowly damage the secretory cells beyond the point where normal function or regeneration is possible, and the abnormal sugar responses result.

Diabetes may be prevented by the long-term ingestion of daily optimal amounts of ascorbic acid to keep dehydroascorbic acid-ascorbic acid ratios at a minimum. The long-term research needed to prove or disprove this thesis will be expensive, but preventing diabetes or hypoglycemia in millions of cases would certainly be worth all the costs.

24

CHEMICAL STRESSES — POISONS, TOXINS

One of the main functions of ascorbic acid in the mammalian body is to maintain normalcy under the effects of environmental stresses. To accomplish this, when under stress, most mammals merely produce more ascorbic acid in their liver. Stress covers a wide variety of conditions, and in this chapter we will discuss chemical stresses. The chemical stresses include such hazards to which we are exposed by contact, breathing, eating, and smoking; attacks by poisonous insects and reptiles; and the highly poisonous toxins of bacterial growth and infection. The amount of work expended over the past forty years on the use of ascorbic acid to counteract the bad effects of chemical stresses is voluminous and it is again impossible to completely cover the field. Even for a brief introduction to this subject, we must subdivide the topic. First, let us see what medical literature reveals about inorganic poisons.

Inorganic Poisons

The majority of the inorganic chemical hazards consist of the poisonous metals, such as the mercury in the seafood we eat, the lead in the paint chips killing ghetto children, the hazardous industrial metals, and the pharmaceutical metals like arsenic.

Mercury. In 1951, Vauthey showed that a certain dose of mercury cyanide injected into guinea pigs killed 100 percent of the animals within 1 hour. If, prior to this mercury injection, he kept his guinea pigs on megascorbic levels of ascorbic acid (equivalent to 35 grams a day for a human weighing 70 kilograms or 154 pounds), 40 percent survived the mercury poisoning. A similar protective effect against bichloride of mercury had been found ten years earlier by Mavin in Argentina. This was further confirmed, in 1964, by Mokranjac and Petrovic. Certain mercury compounds are used in medicine, such as diuretics (to reduce body fluids), which produce toxic reactions in patients. Chapman and Shaffer, in 1947, showed that the toxicity of certain mercurial diuretics could be reduced by prior or simultaneous administration of ascorbic acid. They also reported that in cardiac failure patients, a dose of only 150 milligrams of ascorbic acid increased the diuretic action by 50 percent. Further work on ascorbic acid and the mercurial diuretics was reported by Ruskin and Ruskin in 1952 (1).

Lead. In the 1939 report of a study of 400 workers in a large industrial plant, where exposure to lead hazards was great, Holmes and coworkers observed that the symptoms of chronic lead poisoning resembled subclinical scurvy. As an experiment, they used a group of seventeen people with chronic lead poisoning and gave them 100 milligrams of ascorbic acid daily. Within a week or less: "Most of the men enjoyed normal sleep, lost the irritability and nervousness so common with high calcium treatment of lead poisoning, enjoyed their food more and no longer had the tremors. Several cases of leukopenia [low white cell blood counts] . . . were cured by the ascorbic acid treatment."

Marchmont-Robinson, in 1941, working with 303 employees of an automobile body plant, where lead exposure was high due to the practice of soldering the seams with lead-containing solder and grinding it to a smooth finish, exposed workers to both lead fumes and lead dust. Beginning in June 1939, each worker was given two sticks of gum containing 50 milligrams of ascorbic acid at lunch. The author states, "This study confirms the contention of Holmes that vitamin C (ascorbic acid) has a detoxifying action on lead in the human body." He concludes with the statement, "The routine administration of 50 milligrams of ascorbic acid daily appears to protect workers exposed to lead dust against the usual effects of chronic absorption" (2).

In tests on animals, Pillemer et al. (2) reported tests on guinea pigs poisoned with massive doses of lead carbonate (an old-time white paint pigment) and fed different levels of ascorbic acid. In discussing "paralysis, convulsions, and death," the report states:

> Here the beneficial effects of a high ascorbic acid intake were striking and appear to be unequivocal. In both experiments only two of the twenty-six guinea pigs on the vitamin C regime developed clear-cut spasticities or paralysis, and none of the pigs died of lead poisoning during the period of observation. On the other hand, eighteen of the forty-four animals on the low ascorbic acid intake developed some form of neuroplumbism and twelve died of typical lead poisoning.

The so-called high and low intakes were respectively 50 milligrams and 2.5 milligrams per kilogram of body weight, assuming the guinea pigs weighed about 400 grams (the authors did not report the guinea pig weights). On this basis the daily ascorbic acid intakes for an adult human for their "high" successful series would be 3,500 milligrams and for their "low" ineffectual series, 155 milligrams. But even this ineffectual level is more than twice the current daily recommended allowance for man.

At this point, we will discuss the short note appearing in 1940 in which Dannenberg et al. (2) conclude, "Extremely large doses of ascorbic acid were without effect in the treatment of lead intoxication in a child aged twenty-seven months." From the time the child was fifteen months old, it had eaten wood, paper, and painted articles. When first seen it was a very sick, thirty-six-pound, twenty-seven-month-old boy and a diagnosis was made of chronic lead poisoning and lead encephalosis. For seventeen days the little boy was given 100 milligrams daily of ascorbic acid in divided doses and a daily injection of 250 milligrams ascorbic acid, for a total of 350 milligrams per day. For perspective, this calculates only to about 1.5 grams a day based on a 150-pound adult. A blood examination showed the lead content to be over twelve times higher than normal. After seventeen days, the child showed no improvement and was taken off the "high" ascorbic acid and other therapy was substituted which still included 50 milligrams of ascorbic acid a day. The child was discharged eighty-three days after admission, but still not completely free of the after-effects of the lead intoxication. It is likely in this case that the lead poisoning was so severe that the so-called extremely large doses of ascorbic acid were insufficient to cope with the problem. The fact that the child did not die in the first few weeks after hospitalization and slowly recuperated is probably an unrecognized tribute to the value of ascorbic acid.

In 1963, Gontzea and coworkers (2) studied the blood ascorbic acid levels in long-term workers in a lead-storage battery plant. The blood levels were found to be low and they concluded that persons exposed to lead require larger intakes of ascorbic acid to avoid subclinical scurvy.

In further tests on animals, three Chinese workers, W. Han-Wen et al., kept a hundred tadpoles in water with high lead content for twenty-four hours and eight died. The living tadpoles were divided into tanks containing plain water as a control and plain water containing 31 mg % of ascorbic acid. Six days later, all the tadpoles in the ascorbic acid treated water were alive, while 88 percent in the plain water had died. Uzbekov, in 1960, reported the results of his tests on lead-poisoned rabbits using ascorbic acid and cysteine. He concluded that this combination should not only be used in the treatment of lead poisoning but also as an antidote (2).

Arsenic.   In the early 1940s, various arsenical compounds were in current use for the treatment of syphilis. These compounds produced toxic reactions in the patients and many papers were published showing the detoxifying properties of ascorbic acid when used in combination with these arsenical drugs. Typical are the reports of McChesney and associates, and Abt, in 1942; Lahiri, in 1943; and McChesney, in 1945. Lahiri states, "The administration of vitamin C is the safest way of avoiding arsenical intolerance in antisyphilitic therapy." In 1962, Marocco and E. Rigotti showed that ascorbic acid prevented kidney damage in arsenic poisoning (3).

Chromium and Gold.   The recent work of Samitz and coworkers (4) has shown that ascorbic acid can be used to prevent chromium poisoning and chrome ulcers in industry. Gold salts are used medicinally and have toxic actions on the patient which can be prevented with ascorbic acid, as was shown in Brazil in 1937 and 1940 (5).

In the above review we have covered the poisonous metals (mercury, lead, chromium, and gold) and a nonmetal (arsenic). In each case, ascorbic acid was shown to counteract the poisonous effects. Yet all this suggestive work has apparently been ignored, particularly in two current serious problems: first, the deaths or long-term damage of children from eating paint chips containing lead, and second, exposure to high mercury levels in certain seafoods.

Organic Poisons

Benzene Poisoning. Benzene is a component in various chemical manufacturing processes, such as DDT production, and workers may be exposed to vapors from this volatile ingredient. Many papers, dating back to 1937, have been published showing that exposure to benzene depletes the body of ascorbic acid, that this brings on a state of subclinical scurvy, and that the administration of ascorbic acid helps prevent and alleviate the symptoms of chronic benzene exposure. The 1965 paper by Lurie gives an excellent review and many references to the early literature. Lurie was able to eliminate chronic benzene poisoning among the workers in a South African chemical plant by seeing to it that they received some ascorbic acid in a daily ration of orange juice. In the Czech paper by Thiele, in 1964, he states the chronic benzene poisoning causes, " . . . vitamin C deficiency without signs of scurvy, [and] toxic damage of the capillaries and excessive bleeding." These latter symptoms are characteristic of prolonged deprivation of ascorbic acid. Forssman and Frykholm, in 1947, reported from Stockholm that, "exposure to benzene creates an increased need of vitamin C and that an extra supply of vitamin C gives increased resistance to the effects of benzene." A Russian paper by Filipov appeared which showed that rats reacted to DDT injections by producing more ascorbic acid. This would indicate that ascorbic acid might be useful in the treatment of DDT poisoning in man and other animals; however, no further work in this critical area was noted (6).

Drugs. The effectiveness of drugs in therapy is limited by their toxic actions on the body. The dosages employed are a compromise between their therapeutic effect and their poisonous effect. Ascorbic acid has long been known to detoxify the poisonous effects of various drugs and to potentiate their therapeutic effects.

The highly poisonous convulsive drug, strychnine, is rendered harmless with ascorbic acid as shown by Dey (7) in 1965 and 1967. All of his mice died when injected with 2 milligrams per kilogram of body weight of strychnine, whereas if the mice were first injected with ascorbic acid 15 minutes before administration of strychnine, they did not die. With ascorbic acid at 100 milligrams per kilogram of body weight, there was 60 percent survival; with 1,000 milligrams per kilogram of body weight, none of the poisoned animals died. For a 70-kilogram animal, the size of a human adult, this would be equivalent to 7 grams and 70 grams of ascorbic acid respectively. Dey also pointed out that his observations might be useful in the treatment of tetanus (lockjaw), which we will discuss later.

In 1959, Schulteiss and Tarai (7) suggested the use of ascorbic acid to avoid the harmful side effects of digitalis therapy of heart disease in the aged. Ascorbic acid reduces the toxicity and side reactions of the sulfa drugs. The toxic effects of aspirin are alleviated by ascorbic acid. Too much vitamin A induces a scurvylike syndrome which is promptly relieved with ascorbic acid as shown by Vedder and Rosenberg in 1938 (8).

In acute poisoning by barbiturates, a 1965 Chinese paper (9) showed that intravenous administration of large doses of ascorbic acid had a therapeutic effect on relieving the depression of the central nervous system caused by the drug. It increased the blood pressure and respiration, and produced more forceful heartbeats. Ten years earlier Klenner reported on his successful treatment of barbiturate poisoning by injecting 54 grams of ascorbic acid on the first day.

A 1960 paper by Ghione (9), from the University of Rome, reported that ascorbic acid at 100 milligrams per kilogram of body weight attenuated and abolished the effects of morphine in rats. With the narcotics problem among our young people reaching such vast proportions, it is a sorry commentary that these observations and others on the efficacy of ascorbic acid have not been the basis of a crash research program to help solve some of the addiction problems. Most addicts and smokers of marijuana are probably in a severe state of subclinical scurvy. It may be possible to utilize megascorbic levels to aid in the treatment of addiction and to relieve the drug withdrawal symptoms. By relieving the subclinical scurvy and maintaining their health at a higher level, it may serve to prevent backsliding to the drugs. We will never know unless the appropriate research is conducted.

A paper on anesthesia and ascorbic acid, in the literature since 1944, should have elicited wide responses in surgery. Beyer and coworkers (10) found that the use of anesthetics had a profound influence on the blood levels of ascorbic acid in dogs. They also found that nonscorbutic, ascorbic acid-deprived guinea pigs became anesthetized sooner and deeper. Recovery was slower and the guinea pigs showed more prolonged toxic aftereffects than animals with adequate ascorbic acid. In one test using chloroform, the acid-deficient animals died from respiratory arrest under conditions which only induced light anesthesia in the ascorbic acid-protected group. I wonder whether in the last twenty-five years any further tests were made to explore these observations and if any hospitals bother to check the ascorbic acid adequacy of their patients before subjecting them to anesthesia? Further exploration may improve the chances for patients undergoing surgery.

Bacterial Toxins.   The toxins are a group of poisons of protein-like nature which may be produced by certain pathogenic bacteria, by insects such as spiders and scorpions, and by poisonous snakes. We will discuss the bacterial toxins first.

The toxins of certain disease-producing bacteria are among the most poisonous substances known. The symptoms and morbidity of the disease are due not so much to the presence of these bacteria, but to the toxins they produce. Much work was expended in the 1930s on the diphtheria toxin and its inactivation by ascorbic acid, but since diphtheria is no longer much of a problem, we will start our discussion with the more important tetanus toxin and its consequent disease, lockjaw.

Tetanus.   Every time you suffer a deep cut, you are a potential victim of the serious, life-threatening disease, tetanus. The spores of the germ *Clostridium tetani* have a wide distribution and are especially abundant in the soil. The germs are anaerobes and cannot grow in the presence of air. Because of this, they only infect deep cuts out of contact with air. The usual treatment is to give a prophylactic injection of tetanus toxoid or antitoxin.

According to Bytchenko of the World Health Organization, tetanus has killed more than a million people in the last ten years, "killing more than smallpox, rabies, plague, anthrax, and polio, yet it receives less attention by public health authorities and medical science than any of these."

If the disease develops in spite of precautions, the patient is in trouble. Current treatment is nearly as bad as the disease itself. There is definite need for an improved therapy and ascorbic acid may be the basis for it if only the research would be conducted.

The 1966 paper by Dey (11) reports on tests with groups of animals given the same amount of tetanus toxin. In the first group given the toxin alone, all animals perished in 47 to 65 hours. The second group, in which ascorbic acid was given (1 gram per kilogram of body weight) at the same time, and then twice daily for three days, all animals survived and only very mild symptoms appeared. Animals of the third group received the ascorbic acid for three days prior to the toxin inoculation and then for three days after. All these animals not only survived, but did not show any symptoms of the poisoning. A fourth group was comprised of animals given the toxin, and the ascorbic acid was withheld until the tetanic symptoms appeared, usually sixteen to twenty-six hours later. They were then inoculated with ascorbic acid (1 gram per kilogram of body weight) twice daily for three days. The ascorbic acid prevented the spread of the symptoms and they all survived. In the fifth group, the ascorbic acid administration was further delayed for forty to forty-seven hours until there were marked symptoms of the disease and all the animals survived. Here is the nucleus of successful results which should have initiated wide-scale research into a disease for which modern medicine has failed to produce an effective treatment. The dosages used by Dey, if scaled up to the size of a human adult of 70-kilogram weight, are equivalent to 140 grams a day. Some will regard this amount as a heroic measure, but it is not far from the 70 grams a day used intravenously for reducing the intraocular pressure in human glaucoma. Further research would indicate the proper dose to be used.

It is of further interest and importance that Klenner, in 1954, reported on the successful treatment of tetanus with massive doses of ascorbic acid. Even long before, in 1938, we find that Nitzesco and coworkers reported inactivating tetanus toxin with ascorbic acid. The details of the needed research will be discussed after we look into the related problem of botulism (11)

Botulism.   Botulism is a deadly type of food poisoning caused by the ingestion of the toxins produced in foods by the growth of the bacteria, *Clostridium botulinum.* This is a germ closely related to the one causing tetanus and grows in nonacid foods in the absence of air. Improperly preserved packaged foods are the main source of this toxin. The onset of the symptoms is abrupt and the mortality may be as high as 65 percent. Five different types of botulinus toxins have been identified, each one requiring its own antiserum for treatment of the disease. The results of treatment with the antiserum are disappointing once the symptoms appear, but the treatment may be effective if applied before the onset of symptoms. Clearly, present therapy is rather primitive and a more effective treatment is needed. The detoxicating powers of ascorbic acid are well known and its action on increasing the survival of animals treated with many related bacterial toxins was reported in 1938 by Buller-Souto and Lima (12). In view of this, it is indeed surprising that use of ascorbic acid as a possible means of therapy and survival in botulism has not been further explored over the past three decades.

Research should be immediately initiated because the problem is pressing and more lives will be lost the longer it is delayed.

The research on tetanus, botulism, and other important bacterial toxins could be combined in initial experiments on guinea pigs and monkeys. Inoculating them with lethal amounts of the toxins and determining the correct amount of ascorbic acid (as sodium ascorbate and administered intravenously) required to permit survival and eliminate the symptoms of these intoxications could be the first step. The amounts used will be in the megascorbic range as established by Dey and Klenner (11).

Snakebite.   There are about 2,500 species of snakes throughout the world and about 10 percent are venomous. This minority causes about 30,000 to 40,000 deaths each year, mostly in Asia. In the United States, about 7,000 people are bitten annually, of which about 40 to 60 percent are children and young adults. The regions of highest incidence are the southern and western states and in the period from 1950 to 1959 there were 158 snakebite deaths in this country. The usual treatment consists of supportive measures and injection of antivenin. It is necessary to identify the snake involved in order to obtain the correct type of antivenin since they are highly specific. For instance, the antivenin for the pit vipers is not recommended for the coral snakes. Since time is of the essence in treating a snakebite, a general treatment based on a more widely available material than antivenin and one not limited by the high specificity for certain snakes would be highly desirable.

There have appeared suggestive reports on the use of ascorbic acid for treating snakebites which have never been properly explored. In 1938, Nitzesco et al. (11) showed that ascorbic acid when mixed with cobra venom rendered it harmless. Guinea pigs injected with the cobra venom were all dead in two to three hours, while those injected with the venom-ascorbic acid mixture, not only all survived, but did not even show any of the snakebite symptoms. They also emphasized the importance of high dosages. With 25 milligrams of ascorbic acid, all the animals survived; with 10 milligrams, the guinea pigs survived for a while, but eventually died; and with 5 milligrams there was no beneficial effect.

A 1947 paper from a Bogotá, Colombia, oil company hospital (13) describes the dramatic emergency treatment of three snakebite cases where the biting snakes were not identified. The victims were first given the local treatment of incision of the wound, suction and tourniquet plus the oral administration of orange or lemon juice. They injected 2 grams of ascorbic acid intravenously every 3 hours. The author, Dr. Perdomo, states that immediately after the first injection of ascorbic acid a very favorable response was noted and, after subsequent injections, there was a complete elimination of all symptoms. The patients were observed up to a week later and showed no general or local complications. A plea was made for more research.

In a 1943 paper from India, Kahn (13) reported that ascorbic acid was ineffective for preventing death in dogs injected with cobra venom. On examination of his experimental conditions, we find that he used only one injection of ascorbic acid to counteract the lethal dose of cobra venom. This dose amounted to only 70 to 140 milligrams of ascorbic acid per kilogram of body weight. Dey (11) required 1,000 to 2,000 milligrams of ascorbic acid per kilogram of body weight to counteract the lethal effects of tetanus toxin. In his dogs Kahn used less than 1/3 to 2/3 of the ascorbic acid dosage employed by Perdomo in humans and between 1/7 and 1/3 of the dosage suggested by Dey. It is likely that, if Kahn's tests were repeated using higher levels of ascorbic acid, the results would be as successful as the others.

Klenner, in 1953, also indicated the usefulness of ascorbic acid for snakebites. In a recent personal communication, he stated that he has not only successfully treated cases of snakebite in man megascorbically, but also in dogs, which totally contradicts Kahn's remarks. In 1957, he also revealed the usefulness of ascorbic acid in treating black widow spider bites. Similarly McCormick, in 1952, used ascorbic acid in the treatment of scorpion stings (13).

Here we have the basis for a simple and apparently harmless and effective treatment for a wide variety of animal toxins which has been available, but ignored, for many years. Further exploration of these known facts, using a procedure similar to the tests suggested previously for tetanus and botulism, may provide a new, effective, and immediate treatment for snakebites, black widow spider bites, scorpion stings, and serious multiple bee stings by the mere intravenous infusion of sodium ascorbate at megascorbic levels. The groundwork has been laid for further exploratory research.

The above discussions are devoted to the bacterial and animal toxins, but ascorbic acid would probably be as effective against the plant toxins, such as mushroom poisons, as is indicated in the 1939 paper by Holland and Chlosta (14). Still their plea for further research remains unanswered to this very day.

The body has other biochemical pathways of detoxication besides ascorbic acid and the liver is usually referred to as the organ of detoxication. Nature moved the ascorbic acid-synthesizing enzymes into the liver during the evolution of the mammals. The liver thus became a much more efficient organ of detoxication, protected against the tissue-damaging effects of the various poisons which were concentrated in the liver. The protective action of ascorbic acid against liver damage was shown in 1943 by Beyer and again in 1965 by Soliman et al. (15). Additional research might show that long-term prophylactic megascorbic intakes may prevent cirrhosis and fatty degeneration of the liver which occur in those chronically exposed to toxic levels of various materials. One group that might benefit from further work in this area is the large number of alcoholics who eventually suffer from liver damage and cirrhosis.

25

PHYSICAL STRESSES

The physical stresses include exposure to heat and cold, physical trauma, burns, noise, high altitude, drowning, and ionizing radiation.

The usual mammalian response to stress is increased secretion of the hormones of the adrenal gland. This increased adrenal activity depletes ascorbic acid from the gland, which normally contains a higher concentration of ascorbic acid than any other body tissue. In mammals which produce their own ascorbic acid, this depletion is rapidly replenished. In the guinea pig, some monkeys, and man, the depletion is made up by robbing the body of its tissue stores of ascorbic acid. If the tissue stores are low, adrenal ascorbic acid may be insufficiently restored and the normal adrenal hormonal response to continued stress may become inadequate.

In 1952, Pirani (1) published a review of the work of the first twenty years of the ascorbic acid era. In the bibliography there were 242 references on the relationship of ascorbic acid to stress phenomena. Here, again, we are confronted with a mass of literature from which we can select only a few. The conclusion reached in this review was that under normal conditions, the tissue stores are adequate to cope with acute stress. However, during severe chronic stress, especially after traumatic injuries or burns, and during protracted stimulation of the adrenal cortex, the administration of ascorbic acid is indicated.

Heat and Burns

In a paper on "artificial fever" in which guinea pigs and human subjects were exposed to high environmental temperatures, Zook and Sharpless, in 1938, showed that high temperature exposure accelerates the destruction of ascorbic acid and increases the physiological need for it. Twenty-one years later, Thompson and coworkers confirmed this on women living in southern Arizona. They demonstrated that the rate of depletion of ascorbic acid in blood serum was significantly higher in summer than in winter. The basal metabolism, in a majority of their subjects, also diminished significantly in the summer. They stated, "It is apparent that ascorbic acid metabolism was altered in some manner due to increased requirement or destruction " (2).

In 1944, a paper by Henschel and coworkers (2) was published on *short-term* tests on the ability to work in hot environments. The subjects had been exposed to high temperatures from three hours to four days, under rigidly controlled environmental, dietary, and work conditions. Some of the subjects had been given 500 milligrams of ascorbic acid a day. This work was summarized as having "failed to demonstrate any significant advantage for men receiving supplements of ascorbic acid."

Then along in 1948 came the report by Weaver (2) on the prevention of heat prostration describing *long-term* tests on workers in a Virginia rayon plant who had been exposed to high temperatures and humidities. Weaver found that he was able to eliminate heat prostration in the employees by the daily administration of only 100 milligrams of ascorbic acid. Before instituting this regimen in 1938, there had been twenty-seven cases of heat prostration; in the following 9 years not a single case was reported in the group taking the daily 100 milligrams. During the discussion following the presentation of this paper, Dr. Weaver described the case of heat prostration in a subcontractor who was brought to his medical department at 3 p.m. in collapse and cyanotic. He administered 500 milligrams of ascorbic acid intravenously and by 6 P.M. the man was able to walk to his car and return home. He was back on his job the next day.

A similar test, conducted in the high temperatures near the furnaces of a steel plant, on combinations of salt tablets with vitamins, failed to show any benefits from the vitamins. In this study, Shoudy and Collings administered even less ascorbic acid than the marginal levels used by Weaver. In any further clinical work conducted in this area, megascorbic levels of sodium ascorbate should be used. Sufficient sodium ascorbate must be available to maintain homeostasis under the severe heat stresses. Weaver used only about 1 milligram per kilogram of body weight. Agarkov reported in 1962 that 15 milligrams per kilogram of body weight improved the heat resistance of rats (2). Further studies are required to assess the proper usage of ascorbic acid in heat stress.

The use of ascorbic acid in the treatment of severe burns has been neglected, even after Klasson (3) published his dramatic results in 1951. His basic procedure might have eliminated suffering and saved the lives of many fire victims over the past twenty years if it had been more widely used. Klasson reported on sixty-two burn cases from a variety of causes such as hot water, hot grease, gasoline explosions, and chemical agents. He used ascorbic acid topically, by mouth, and intravenously. He applied a 1 percent ascorbic acid solution in 0.9 percent salt solution or a 2 percent ascorbic acid ointment in a water-soluble base directly to the burned area. When these were applied, there was immediate relief from pain, which permitted a reduction in the morphine given the victims. Spraying the throat or gargling with 1 percent ascorbic acid in normal saline solution, rapidly alleviated the hoarseness and pain caused by swallowing smoke. In addition, Klasson gave up to 2,000 milligrams of ascorbic acid a day by mouth or intravenously and at "no time were deleterious effects from the drug observed." In severe burn cases, there is usually a suppression of urine and Klasson found the ascorbic acid treatment maintained the urinary output at normal levels. He summarized his study by stating that ascorbic acid alleviates pain, hastens healing, combats the accumulation of toxic protein metabolites in severe burn cases, and reduces the time needed before skin grafting.

Klenner (4), in 1971, stated he had found the "secret" for

reducing pain and infection from severe burns, preventing toxemia and promoting healing. This method is summarized in the following five steps: 1. The patient is kept unclothed without dressings in a warmed cradle. 2. A 3 percent solution of ascorbic acid is sprayed over the entire burned area every two to four hours for about five days. 3. Vitamin A and D ointment is then alternated with the 3 percent ascorbic acid spray. 4. Megascorbic doses are administered by mouth and vein of 500 milligrams of ascorbic acid per kilogram body weight as sodium ascorbate (35 grams for a 70-kilogram adult) every eight hours (105 grams a day) for the first several days, then at twelve-hour intervals (1 gram calcium gluconate is given daily to replace calcium lost in body fluids). 5. Supportive treatment is given. ·

What more suggestive and promising leads are required to start a program of research to explore a new treatment for burns to replace the rather primitive methods now used? Klasson cites fifteen references from the medical literature, dating back to 1936, which led him to try ascorbic acid. Later work (5) showed the profound influence of burns on the ascorbic acid metabolism, but no group bothered to conduct the large-scale crucial clinical trials using ascorbic acid or sodium ascorbate at megascorbic levels (topically, orally, and intravenously), to develop an improved therapy.

Cold

There is a considerable medical literature on cold temperatures and their effect on the ascorbic acid in the body. Outstanding are the investigations of the Canadian Dugal and coworkers, starting in 1947, continuing for many years, and summarized in 1961. In their 1947 paper (6), they reported that rats, which were exposed for long periods to freezing temperatures, but which were able to adjust to these low temperatures, had large increases in the ascorbic acid levels of their body tissues; whereas, those rats unable to adjust to the cold environment had decreased levels. They concluded that maintenance of life at low temperatures requires large quantities of ascorbic acid. This was further confirmed with tests on guinea pigs.

In long-term tests on monkeys reported in 1952, Dugal and Fortier (6) found that among monkeys exposed for six months to cold temperatures (50°F) and then subjected to subfreezing temperatures (-4°F) those given 325 milligrams of ascorbic acid daily for the six-month period were far more resistant to the intense cold than those given only 25 milligrams a day. Since their monkeys weighed about 12.5 pounds, this calculates to 4,000 milligrams, or 4 grams, a day based on the weight of a human adult (70 kilograms) for the cold-resistant group and 300 milligrams daily for the group showing no resistance.

No tests have been conducted to determine if the resistance of humans to cold temperatures could be improved using 4 grams or more of ascorbic acid. One short-term test (thirteen days) on soldiers, reported in 1954, employed only 525 milligrams of ascorbic acid a day in one group and 25 milligrams in another. Both groups were exposed to cold temperatures on survival rations. The group on the high, but still marginal levels of 525 milligrams, showed improved resistance to the cold and a large decrease in foot troubles over the 25-milligram group. In another short-term test reported, in 1946, Glickman and coworkers broadly concluded that the results of their experiment indicated clearly that the ability of men to withstand the damaging effects of repeated exposures to cold environments cannot be appreciably enhanced by giving "excessive" doses of ascorbic acid or other vitamins above the amounts required for adequate nutrition. However, their idea of an "excessive" dose of ascorbic acid was 200 milligrams a day, which had been shown to be ineffective in the monkey experiments previously mentioned (6). We cannot say, at this point, whether the megascorbic levels will improve human resistance to cold or not, but if further tests are to be conducted, they should use at least the levels found successful in monkeys. There are millions of people suffering each year from the effects of winter cold who may benefit if these tests yield successful results.

Physical Trauma

Ungar (7), a member of the Free French Forces studying wound ballistics, provided information of vital importance which might have saved the lives of thousands of soldiers and auto accident victims if it had been properly followed up. The purpose of his study was to relate the degree of trauma expressed in terms of physical energy with the severity of shock as estimated by mortality. Ungar took anesthetized guinea pigs and dropped known weights from different heights onto the animals and found there was a definite relationship between transmitted energy and tissue damage and mortality. The startling fact brought out by his research was that in guinea pigs subjected to the dropped weights, which ordinarily would kill 100 percent of the animals, these animals would always survive if given an injection of ascorbic acid in doses above 100 milligrams per kilogram of body weight shortly after the trauma. His injection dosage calculates to over 7 grams of ascorbic acid, based on a 70-kilogram body weight. The prompt administration of this amount or more of ascorbic acid on the battlefield to wounded soldiers or to auto accident victims at the scene may prevent shock and insure survival until they reach a hospital. You might well ask how it is possible for such an important observation to lay dormant for 30 years.

Bone Fracture

The 1946 paper by Andreae and Browne (7) showed that in man, both burn and bone fracture trauma produce rapid decreases of ascorbic acid in the whole blood and the white blood cells.

A 1962 paper from the Soviet Union by Merezhinskii (7) reported tests on guinea pigs with bone fractures. Merezhinskii showed that the daily administration of 40 milligrams of ascorbic acid was sufficient to correct for the ascorbic acid losses due to the trauma but 10 milligrams were not. He found that the recovery from bone fractures was considerably shortened when large doses of ascorbic acid were given. His successful 40-milligram dose, when scaled up to a 150-pound body weight, amounts to the daily intake of about 9 grams of ascorbic acid, while his inadequate 10-milligram dose is equivalent to 2.3 grams a day.

High Altitude

Exposure to high altitudes is a severe form of stress because the rarefied atmosphere induces oxygen deprivation, known as hypoxia. Hypoxia is a lack of the proper levels of oxygen in the blood and tissues. Severe hypoxia can be induced in the body by means other than high altitude, such as drowning. Our discussion of high altitudes will also apply to these other conditions.

If people are transported from sea level to high mountainous altitudes, there is a chance that they will develop acute mountain sickness before they become accustomed to the great heights. The disease is called *soroche* in the Andes and probably has many other local names in various mountain areas. The air we breathe contains about 20 percent oxygen at sea level but only about 15 percent at about 15,000 feet. High altitude was also a problem in aviation before the advent of the pressurized cabin.

As long ago as 1938 it was perceived that ascorbic acid increases the altitude tolerance of ski troops and rabbits. Peterson, in 1941, showed that mice injected with ascorbic acid were able to withstand repeated exposure to air pressures that were 1/6 normal, while their untreated companions succumbed. Krasno and coworkers showed, in 1950, using human subjects repeatedly exposed to 18,000-foot altitude conditions, increased utilization of ascorbic acid with consequent depletion. This was confirmed in guinea pigs exposed to the same high altitudes, with the animals manifesting abnormally low levels of tissue ascorbic acid. In a 1959 paper from Yugoslavia, Wesley and coworkers reported that in guinea pigs exposed for one hour to low air pressures equivalent to a 30,-000-foot height, there was a drop in ascorbic acid levels and a substantial increase in the more toxic dehydroascorbic acid levels. This was also confirmed in dogs; and tests were made on men who responded similarly to the hypoxia, depending upon the intensity and duration of exposure (8).

Even with this extensive background of suggestive research, I was unable to find anyone who was inspired to prevent altitude sickness or the bad effects of hypoxia by the administration of high levels of ascorbic acid. The closest to a test of this nature was reported by Brooks (8), in 1948, using the dyestuff, methylene blue. She found that if people who normally suffered from altitude sickness were given 0.2 grams of the methylene blue before ascending to about 15,000 feet in a four-hour automobile trip, they no longer became ill. Also, untreated subjects who became ill with headache and nausea at 10,000 feet, if given 0.1 gram of methylene blue, were free of the symptoms within an hour. Methylene blue and ascorbic acid are both members of oxidation-reduction systems and should have similar therapeutic actions. Anything methylene blue can do, ascorbic acid should do better. The diuretic effect of ascorbic acid should also help relieve the pulmonary edema that develops at high altitudes. It is time now for the necessary further clinical work, since hypoxia is a widespread problem much beyond altitude sickness. The results obtained would be important in the treatment of the hypoxia of nonfatal drownings, of infants during birth, during anesthesia in surgery, in prolonged surgical procedures, and in suffocation cases, to prevent brain damage.

Radiation

Exposure to radiation is an extremely stressful situation for the living organism. The term "radiation" includes ultraviolet rays, X rays, gamma rays, and other ionizing radiation in the radiant-energy spectrum. The dangers of exposure to X rays have been recognized in recent years and the radiation casualties of the atom bombings are proof of the hazards. Exposure to radiation, as an occupational hazard for physicians specializing in radiology, has had a life-shortening effect and has increased susceptibility to disease, as compared to physicians in other specialties (9).

There have been numerous papers published showing that exposure to X rays lowers the levels of ascorbic acid in the body: Kretzschmer et al., in 1947; Monier and Weiss, in 1952; Hochman et al. and Oster et al., in 1953; Dolgova, in 1962; and many other papers from the Soviet Union from 1963 on (10). In general, these papers indicate that in guinea pigs, which cannot synthesize their own ascorbic acid under stress, there are decreases of ascorbic acid in the blood and tissues after irradiation. Animals, such as rats and rabbits, that produce ascorbic acid in their livers under stress usually suffer an initial drop in their ascorbic acid level which rises after the liver has had a chance to replace the lost ascorbic acid. If the irradiation is severe enough to interfere with the synthesis of ascorbic acid, the losses remain.

The use of ascorbic acid as a protection against the unfavorable effects of radiation goes back many years and, in spite of the fact that the investigators used pitifully small doses of ascorbic acid, many reported good results. Carrie and Schnettler, in 1939, using only 200 milligrams a day of ascorbic acid, reported good results and recommended it as the medication of choice. They were able to prevent the leukopenia (reduction of white blood cells in the blood) induced by exposure to X rays. This was confirmed by Clausen, in 1942, who prevented the leukopenia in ten stomach-cancer patients treated with X rays by giving them a daily injection of 500 milligrams of ascorbic acid. Wallace, in 1941, injected only 50 milligrams of ascorbic acid daily and was able to report that it prevented many general symptoms of radiation sickness and almost entirely eliminated the severe nausea and vomiting, but it did not prevent the intestinal changes due to the heavy pelvic X-ray treatments administered (11).

Kalnins, from Sweden, who published many other papers in this area, reported in 1953 that the X-ray lesions of guinea pigs given 50 milligrams a day of ascorbic acid were much better protected against the damaging radiation effects than those given only 1 milligram a day. He thought that the large doses of ascorbic acid acted as detoxicants for the histaminelike bodies or the leukotoxins developed in the irradiated tissue. Yusipov, from the Soviet Union, in two short papers reporting tests in 1959 on rabbits and rats that did not specify the dosages of ascorbic acid he used, indicated that if ascorbic acid was given before the irradiation, it exerted an unfavorable effect, but if administered afterward it was beneficial. He recommended the use of ascorbic acid in the treatment of acute radiation sickness in the latent period and period of climax. He mentions that the clarification of the role of ascorbic acid in acute radiation sickness is one for the immediate future (11). Several papers have appeared showing the protective effect of ascorbic acid on various bodily enzymes against destruction by ionizing radiation. In the 1965 paper by Shapiro et al. (12), the scientists suggested the comprehensive testing of ascorbic acid as a radiation-protective agent in animals.

Although the usefulness of ascorbic acid has been indicated, the crucial clinical tests, using the higher levels of ascorbic acid, have not been initiated. These long-overdue tests should be started and thoroughly explored.

26

POLLUTION AND SMOKER'S SCURVY

Great effort is being expended to cleanse our environment and there is hope for eventual success in minimizing man-made contamination. There are, however, some areas which may not fully respond, and a complete elimination of pollutants certainly is not likely in the foreseeable future. One area of pollution is the natural background radiation level due to cosmic and other radiation from the sun and outer space. Even when crowds of people congregate they are irradiating themselves and surrounding people with the rays from the radioactive potassium in their bodies. Another segment is in carbon monoxide exposure. While a major source of local carbon monoxide buildup in the atmosphere is due to combustion of fuels, (estimated to produce 200 million tons a year), even if this were completely eliminated, there would still be other sources. Carbon monoxide is produced naturally in the human body at the rate of 0.42 milliliter per hour and a major source of carbon monoxide intoxication is cigarette smoking (1). The oceans are a natural source for carbon monoxide (2) as well as plants (1). The air over the oceans and virgin forests, far from human contamination, would thus never be free of a low, but definite, level of carbon monoxide. Traces of carbon monoxide are even found in stored soft drinks (3). Thus, it would be impossible for one to avoid carbon monoxide altogether.

Measures to lessen direct contamination of the air and soil are being developed, but it may take years for them to take noticeable effect. In the meantime, a supplemental approach to this problem, which is being suggested, is to make the population more resistant to the harmful effects of the pollutants by using ascorbic acid. The previous chapters on the effects of ascorbic acid in combating the various chemical and physical stresses suggest a valid basis for this new approach. The daily administration of a few grams of ascorbic acid may be adequate to increase the resistance of the body to these chronic toxic environmental stresses.

In the case of carbon monoxide toxicity, a 1962 paper from the Soviet Union (3) showed that chronic exposure of guinea pigs to carbon monoxide increased the rate of consumption of and requirement for, ascorbic acid. The effects of chronic carbon monoxide poisoning were counteracted by administering 40 milligrams of ascorbic acid daily. For a 300-gram guinea pig, 40 milligrams are equivalent to 9,000 milligrams (9 grams) for a 150-pound body weight. In 1955, Klenner (3) noted that the treatment of choice for carbon monoxide poisoning, both acute and chronic, was ascorbic acid. Two other papers need to be mentioned in this discussion, one appearing as far back as 1938 and the other in 1958. Ungar and Bolgert (4) showed that ascorbic acid would protect guinea pigs against death from exposure to high concentrations of hydrochloric acid vapor, nitric oxide, and other vapors. To be effective, however, it was necessary to give *not less* than 500 milligrams per kilogram of body weight, which is equivalent to about 35,000 milligrams for a 150-pound body weight. Ozone, a necessary constituent of the upper atmosphere and a contaminant produced in the air we breathe under certain conditions, is a toxic oxidizing substance. Mittler (4), in 1958, reported that a single injection of ascorbic acid into mice before exposing them, for 3 hours, to air containing an ozone level of 8 to 25 parts per million, provided a higher rate of survival than among untreated mice.

Will the agencies now so concerned with our external environment also be concerned with our individual internal environment and implement research on the use of ascorbic acid to combat environmental hazards?

Smoking

Smoking is an intense form of concentrated individual air pollution. With all the furor about cleaning up the air we breathe, smokers nonchalantly inhale the concentrated smoke from a plug of burning tobacco an inch or two from their face. This smoke contains levels of gaseous pollutants—carbon monoxide, hydrocyanic acid, nitric oxide, sulfur dioxide, and acetonitrile—in much higher concentrations than would ever be permitted in the air we breathe. In addition, the smoke contains finely dispersed carcinogenic tars, poisons such as nicotine, radioactive dust such as polonium-210, and other ingredients. These are deposited on the tissues of the mouth, tongue, pharynx, bronchi, and interior of the nose. We have here a highly irritating form of local chemical stress which depletes the tissues of their stores of ascorbic acid. Research may eventually show that this chronic irritation and depletion are what finally trigger the neoplastic process.

Many reports can be found in the medical literature on the destructive influence of tobacco smoke on the ascorbic acid levels of the body. As far back as 1939, Strauss and Scheer (5) found that smoking produced a constant and marked reduction in the excretion of ascorbic acid, indicating its destruction in the body by smoke constituents. McCormick (5), in 1952, stated:

> In determining the anti-infectious protective dosage of vitamin C there is another factor which is not generally considered. When the vitamin is employed to neutralize toxins of endogenous or exogenous origin, the action is reciprocal in that the vitamin is also neutralized proportionately, leaving less available for physiological needs. To illustrate, the writer has determined by laboratory and clinical tests that the smoking of one cigarette neutralizes in the body approximately 25 milligrams of vitamin C, or the amount in one medium-sized orange. It will thus be seen how difficult it is to meet the bodily requirement of the pack-a-day smoker for even the protective level of vitamin C from dietary sources. It is thus obvious that the steady smoker, who is usually short on his dietary intake as well, requires a much heavier therapeutic dosage of this vitamin than the nonsmoker.

Bourquin and Musmanno (5), in 1953, reported that nicotine,

added to human blood, decreased its ascorbic acid content by 24 to 31 percent. They concluded that larger amounts of ascorbic acid should be taken by habitually heavy smokers.

Venulet, in a series of papers published during 1951 to 1956, as reviewed by Andrzejewski (5), showed that the inhalation of tobacco smoke produced a marked loss of ascorbic acid in animals and man. In 60 medical students, the blood ascorbic acid levels were 1.0 to 1.2 mg % in nonsmokers, and 0.6 to 0.9 mg % in smokers. The nonsmokers who volunteered to smoke six to eight cigarettes a day suffered a significant decrease in serum ascorbic acid levels by the third day. This drop disappeared five days after cessation of the smoking. If the levels in man parallel those found in animals, there is a large decrease for each internal organ. There are considerable differences in the ascorbic acid content found in the milk of smoking and nonsmoking mothers. Maximal differences occur in the spring when the levels average 5.9 mg % in nonsmoking women against 2.1 mg % in smoking women. Venulet concluded that smoking is involved in the pathogenesis of certain widespread disorders such as scurvy, gastric ulcer, and cardiovascular disease. Apart from difficulties arising from ascorbic acid depletion, smoking lowers the general bodily resistance to disease.

Goyanna (5), in 1955, in a paper entitled "Tobacco and Vitamin C" thoroughly indicts tobacco smoking for its destructive action on the body's ascorbic acid. He showed that in heavy smokers, ascorbic acid is destroyed and no longer excreted in the urine. He described the many functions of ascorbic acid in the body including its role in detoxicating poisons. In his concluding paragraph he states, "The salvation of the smoker may be in this vitamin."

In 1960, Dietrich and Büchner (5), demonstrated lowered blood plasma ascorbic acid levels in smokers and concluded that smokers exhibit a vitamin C deficiency compared to nonsmokers. They advised all smokers to consume an abundance of vitamin C to prevent development of a deficiency.

Durand et al. (5), in 1962, also confirmed that the blood ascorbic acid of smokers is lower than nonsmokers. He gave 1 gram of ascorbic acid a day to pack-and-a-half cigarette smokers and found that the increases in blood ascorbic acid never attained the peak levels shown by nonsmokers. He concluded that there is an ascorbic acid deficiency in smokers. Rupniewska (5), in 1965, also reported a decreased store of ascorbic acid in aged smokers.

Calder, Curtis, and Fore (5), in 1963, indicated that tobacco smoke destroyed vitamin C in solution. They also demonstrated a statistically significant difference in blood plasma ascorbic acid and leukocyte ascorbic acid contents of cigarette smokers and non-smokers. The more cigarettes smoked, the lower were the ascorbic acid blood levels.

A 1968 study by Brook and Grimshaw (5) demonstrated that blood plasma and leukocyte ascorbic acid levels are signficantly lower in men than in women. In nonsmokers, the plasma levels declined with age while the leukocyte levels did not. Cigarette smoking was found to significantly lower both the blood plasma and the leukocyte ascorbic acid concentrations. Heavy smoking had the same effect on the blood plasma ascorbic acid as increasing the chronological age by 40 years.

Pelletier (5), in tests on five smokers and five nonsmokers, as reported in 1968, demonstrated that the ascorbic acid levels of the blood and blood plasma of smokers were about 40 percent that of nonsmokers. On giving his subjects 2 grams of ascorbic acid a day, he found that after continued administration the blood ascorbic acid levels stabilized at approximately the same values for both groups. However, the urinary excretion of ascorbic acid by the smokers never reached the levels excreted by the nonsmokers, which indicated a continuing greater utilization of the ascorbic acid by the smokers. He also made tests on guinea pigs which were fed nicotine for one month in amounts comparable to those consumed by heavy smokers. There was a drop in the blood and tissue ascorbic acid, as compared to guinea pigs fed the same diet without the nicotine, amounting to 49 percent in the adrenal gland, 50 percent in the kidneys, 47 percent in the heart, and 34 percent in the liver.

From all this research work, it should be evident that habitual smokers, unless they take steps to correct the condition, are likely to be in a chronic, subclinical scorbutic state. In this situation, the classical signs of scurvy may not be manifest, but the body is in a state of biochemical scurvy. With this depletion, there is lowered resistance to disease and the biochemical detoxication processes are impaired. I have termed this bodily condition, "Smoker's Scurvy" and a very simple cure for it is—*stop smoking*.

For the numerous hard-core smokers who cannot kick the habit, cigarette manufacturers could institute a program of research to determine if the long-term daily use of ascorbic acid will provide some protection against cancers, emphysema, coronaries, and other diseases which afflict smokers.

Research conducted at Tulane University by Schlegel and coworkers (6), and mentioned previously, prompted Schlegel to recommend the daily use of 1.5 grams of ascorbic acid to prevent the recurrence of bladder cancer in smokers.

27

WOUNDS, BONE FRACTURES, AND SHOCK

It has been known for hundreds of years that wounds will not heal and that healed old wounds and scars reopen in people deprived of ascorbic acid and afflicted with scurvy. Scurvy also weakens the bones and renders them more susceptible to fracture. In the forty years since the discovery of ascorbic acid, there have been so many papers published on the beneficial relationship of ascorbic acid to wound healing, on the improved strength of the scar tissue, and on the faster healing of bone fractures, that it is just impossible to fully review this vast volume of work within a brief chapter. However, the interested reader can refer to the papers presented at the Scientific Conference on vitamin C, held by the New York Academy of Sciences in 1960 (1). The papers by Abt and Schuching, Robertson, Gould, Crandon, Fullmer, and Lee are of particular interest in this connection.

The utilization of ascorbic acid in wound healing is now so well documented that there are many surgeons who routinely provide their patients with 1 or 2 grams of ascorbic acid a day, postoperatively, to aid in their healing and recovery. In spite of the vast number of published papers, it is still not known whether these are the optimal levels for this purpose and whether the patients would benefit from the administration of higher amounts. This should be the subject of further research.

Of particular interest at this point is the recent work of Dr. Steinberg (1), of Jewish Memorial Hospital in New York City, in the successful treatment of gangrene of the legs and feet with sodium ascorbate. In five cases of long-standing gangrene, resistant to other forms of treatment and some scheduled for amputation, the administration of up to 5 grams of sodium ascorbate daily, in addition to other treatment, brought about improvement and healing in a few weeks. These cases of gangrene were caused by arteriosclerotic occlusion, diabetic endarteritis, and polycythemia vera. While the ascorbic acid status of the patients was not determined, it is likely they were suffering from severe chronic subclinical scurvy. Much follow-up work is needed on this promising lead in the treatment of gangrenous lesions.

But even in wound healing, the full potential of ascorbic acid may not be entirely exploited. For instance, there is a critical shortage of hospital beds and all the medical and other facilities necessary to maintain them. Research should be instituted to determine if the daily routine administration of a few grams of ascorbic acid to hospital admissions would hasten their recovery and shorten their hospital stay. Many patients now entering hospitals are already in a prescorbutic state. If their hospital stay could be shortened by 25 percent, it would be equivalent to building and staffing a new facility for every four in existence, at only pennies a day per patient.

Morbidity Index — A New Diagnostic Tool

Another area of medical treatment which requires more investigation is the use of ascorbic acid as a diagnostic and prognostic tool. Blood samples are usually taken from patients and a variety of examinations are made on them. It is rare, however, that a determination of ascorbic acid is ever made on these blood samples. Because of complications in the methodology developed over the years, the determination of ascorbic acid in blood has lost much of its diagnostic value and has fallen into disrepute.

The methods in use during the 1930s determined the true,

"reduced" ascorbic acid in the blood. In 1943, when new procedures were introduced, what was determined was the "total" ascorbic acid, which not only included the "reduced" ascorbic acid but the "oxidized" dehydroascorbic acid and other decomposition products. The actual results obtained by these two different types of methods were not comparable and caused much confusion, which still exists. While it is possible to separately determine the ascorbic acid and the dehydroascorbic acid by either techniques, it was seldom carried out and reported in the research work of the past forty years.

The development of a possible valuable diagnostic tool was delayed for four decades due to a lack of appreciation of the simple physicochemical facts involved. What is needed in these determinations is not the "total" *or* the "reduced" ascorbic acid, but the *ratio* of the two components, ascorbic acid and dehydroascorbic acid. In 1955, Chakrabarti and Banerjee (2), after reviews of the prior work, pointed out the paradox of dehydroascorbic acid which, at low levels, behaves essentially like ascorbic acid in giving protection from or curing scurvy, but is toxic at high levels. They determined both the ascorbic acid and dehydroascorbic acid in the blood of many of their patients. They found that the ascorbic acid levels went down and dehydroascorbic acid levels went up as their patients became sicker and finally died from meningitis, tetanus, pneumonia, and typhoid fever. If the patients survived, the trend was reversed. Hoffer and Osmond (2), in 1963, cited many other references relating to mental stress and mental disease affecting the ascorbic acid blood levels and also first calculated the $\frac{\text{ASCORBIC ACID}}{\text{DEHYDROASCORBIC ACID}}$ ratios which showed some startling statistics. These figures, along with some others which I calculated from another paper (3), are assembled in the following table.

Inspection of the figures on this table shows the inadequacy of "total" ascorbic acid blood levels as a diagnostic measurement. Because of the high dehydroascorbic levels, many of the dead patients had higher "total" levels than the survivors. With many investigators during the past three decades reporting "total" ascorbic acid in their work, it can easily be discerned how the present confusion and lack of confidence in blood ascorbic determinations resulted. The "reduced" ascorbic acid levels are a superior indicator, but most significant is the ratio of $\frac{\text{ASCORBIC ACID}}{\text{DEHYDROASCORBIC ACID}}$, which I term the "morbidity index."

The "normals" had a morbidity index of approximately 15 although an individual taking high levels of ascorbic acid would have even a higher index. Those who were critically sick but survived had a morbidity index of about 1.0, while those who died had much less, 0.3 to 0.5. During convalescence of the survivors, the morbidity index jumped to 3.0 to 5.0.

Morbidity Index as a Prognostic Tool and Index of Survival

Disease and Condition	Number of Patients	"Total" Ascorbic Acid (mg/100 ml)	"Reduced" Ascorbic Acid (AA) (mg/100 ml)	"Oxidized" Ascorbic Acid (DHAA) (mg/100 ml)	Mor-bidity Index AA DHAA
Normal	28	0.93	0.87	0.06	14.0
Meningitis					
died	8	1.22	0.27	0.95	0.3
survived	17	1.04	0.43	0.61	0.7
convalescent	11	0.72	0.53	0.19	2.8
Tetanus					
died	13	1.09	0.36	0.73	0.5
survived	12	0.93	0.52	0.41	1.3
convalescent	12	0.89	0.74	0.15	5.0
Pneumonia					
died	7	0.98	0.30	0.68	0.4
survived	19	0.83	0.43	0.40	1.0
convalescent	15	0.75	0.59	0.16	4.0
Typhoid Fever					
died	4	0.80	0.24	0.56	0.4
survived	19	0.80	0.45	0.35	1.3
convalescent	15	0.83	0.68	0.15	4.5
Chronic tubercular meningitis	17	0.83	0.50	0.33	1.5
Normal	16	0.95	0.89	0.06	14.8
Cholera	21	0.99	0.62	0.37	1.7
Smallpox	16	1.07	0.51	0.56	0.9
Pyogenic Meningitis	16	0.80	0.35	0.45	0.7
Tubercular Meningitis	16	0.92	0.74	0.18	4.2
Gonorrhea	16	0.79	0.53	0.26	2.0
Syphilis	16	0.92	0.74	0.18	4.2

(The figures for the last seven entries in the above table were calculated from the data of Bhaduri et al. (3), while the rest are from Chakrabarti et al. (2).)

There is a logical physicochemical explanation for these variations. Ascorbic acid and dehydroascorbic acid, as explained in earlier chapters, are members of a reversible oxidation-reduction system. The redox potential depends on the relative amounts of each component of the systems. For healthy tissue processes, that ratio must favor high amounts of ascorbic acid and very low levels of dehydroascorbic acid in order to keep the redox potential low. In pathology, the tissue potentials approach more oxidative levels as the disease progresses, and recedes again as the disease clears up.

Incalculable time has been wasted by hundreds of investigators over the past forty years of research work. They were trying to relate ascorbic acid blood levels to a disease process, but did not realize these simple facts and only determined and reported either "total" ascorbic acid or "reduced" ascorbic acid. Much of the confusion during the past four decades is due to this inadequate data.

The value of megascorbic therapy may be in maintaining the redox tissue potentials at the necessary low levels and maintaining the morbidity index in the upper brackets. The constant presence of high ascorbic acid levels may suppress the formation of the toxic dehydroascorbic acid.

Here we have a potentially valuable tool which may aid the physician in determining how sick his patient really is and his chances for survival. Further research should resolve the question of how valuable a tool the morbidity index really can be.

Shock

Shock is a very dangerous condition of general bodily collapse that can rapidly appear as the result of the stresses of severe, traumatic injuries, burns, major surgery, massive hemorrhage, abdominal injury, and dehydration. The fundamental defect in shock is failure of effective blood flow and hence impaired transport of vital materials in the blood to the organs and tissues. This is brought on by increased permeability of the capillaries, resulting in loss of blood plasma into the surrounding tissues. The lowered blood volume, with its increased percentage of blood cellular constituents, is more difficult to pump through the arteries and veins. The volume of blood being pumped from the heart is low and the blood pressure is low. The patient is usually in a state of collapse with a pallid, moist skin and impaired mental faculties. It is necessary to rapidly correct this condition and usually the first measures are to assure proper breathing and replace the blood's volume of fluid.

The use of ascorbic acid in the treatment of shock has been repeatedly suggested in many papers over the past thirty years. These papers include reports not only of successful experiments on laboratory animals, but on case histories on man. There is a perfectly good rationale for this use of ascorbic acid because of its long-known beneficial effects in preventing capillary fragility and the fact that hemorrhage is a characteristic symptom of ascorbic acid depletion. In 1941, in experiments on cats bled of 50 percent of their blood volume, Stewart and coworkers (4) were able to prolong the animals' lives with an intravenous injection of ascorbic acid. Ungar (4), in 1942 and 1943, was able to prevent traumatic shock and death in injured guinea pigs by an injection of ascorbic acid of 100 milligrams or more per kilogram of body weight. In 1943, nearly three decades ago, he noted that particular emphasis should be laid on the possibility of utilizing his observations in the treatment of human traumatic and surgical shock.

Further tests on guinea pigs, reported in 1944 by McDevitt and coworkers (4), showed ascorbic acid increased their resistance to trauma and improved their survival. In studies on eleven human subjects undergoing major surgery they sampled the patients' blood for ascorbic acid determinations before, during, and after the operations. Of the eleven cases, five had subnormal ascorbic acid levels before the operation and eight had levels markedly below normal immediately postoperatively or within twenty-four hours.

Hemorrhagic shock induced in guinea pigs by a standardized bleeding procedure was the subject of a 1946 paper by de-Pasqualini (4). She found that if the guinea pigs were given 200 milligrams of ascorbic acid five minutes before the start of bleeding, it prevented hemorrhagic shock and 94 percent of her eighteen test animals survived, while 90 percent of the seventeen animals not given ascorbic acid died.

Holmes (5), in 1946, discussed the use of ascorbic acid to relieve the increased capillary permeability occurring in shock. He cites the successful results of a group of cooperating surgeons using ascorbic acid to successfully treat surgical shock. Another surgeon used it successfully preoperatively and postoperatively in fifty serious abdominal operations. In approximately 2,000 cases of dental extractions, ascorbic acid was administered thirty to forty-five minutes before the extraction, preventing shock and postoperative weakness. It was also employed in thirty-five cases of mine injuries, in which instances it helped the injured to survive the long trip to the hospital. He also cites the experiences of other cooperating physicians. He noted that there was no question on the value of adequate amounts of ascorbic acid in the maintenance of a healthy condition of the capillary walls and that it may also be useful in combating the anoxia of shock. The highest blood levels of ascorbic acid were reached after two or three hours on oral administration and in three to five minutes when given intravenously.

In 1946, S. M. Levenson and associates (6), reported on the use of ascorbic acid, vitamins B_1, and B_2, and nicotinic acid in severe injury, hemorrhage, and infections in humans. They concluded that their work adds further support to the idea that large doses of these materials may serve a useful purpose in treating acutely ill patients. In 1962, a conference and workshop on hemorrhagic shock was held at the Rockefeller Institute. As reported in *Science* by Simeone (6), Dr. Levenson presented a paper revealing that injured animals suffer from biochemical scurvy. Levenson's claim that ascorbic acid could influence the mortality from hemorrhagic shock was "viewed with skepticism."

In 1947, Zerbini (7) reported on a duodenal ulcer operation where the patient went into postoperative shock. Prompt administration of 2 grams of ascorbic acid, intravenously, pulled him out of the shock within minutes. Continued large dosages of ascorbic acid made the patient's recovery "uneventful." Zerbini noted that his one observation is merely suggestive but that "further studies would obviously seem worthwhile." In the course of tests in eighty surgical operations, Pataky and associates (7) reported in 1957 that they were able to inhibit the passage of plasma through the intact vessel walls, and to control surgical shock with large doses of ascorbic acid. Kashchevskaia (7), in a 1958 paper from the Soviet Union, showed that ascorbic acid is intimately involved in the state of shock.

Strawitz and coworkers (8), using rats to determine the effect of ascorbic acid and methylene blue in hemorrhagic shock, reported in 1958 that both agents significantly reduced the mortality rates and, in addition, ascorbic acid lengthened the survival period.

In 1963, Santomé and Gomez (9), using dogs as experimental animals, checked the earlier work of Sayers et al. on rats in hemorrhagic shock. They found an increase in the blood ascorbic acid levels and a highly significant decrease in the adrenal gland ascorbic acid, in spite of the higher levels in the blood. The higher blood level is likely to be an artifact because the liver rapidly synthesized ascorbic acid under the stress and it poured it into a reduced volume of blood. The low ascorbic acid levels in the adrenal glands are probably a more reliable criteria of the response to the heavy stresses to which the animals were subjected.

In a paper published in 1967, Kocsard-Varo (9) discussed microcirculation (the capillary system), capillary permeability, and ascorbic acid. She made the following interesting observation which involved her in the study of the microcirculation. She found that in nosebleed due to high blood pressure, if a 1–1,000 adrenaline solution were applied to the surface of the nasal mucous membrane or if ascorbic acid were injected individually, the bleeding would continue. However, if they were both done simultaneously, the blood flow stopped "instantaneously, as if one turned off a faucet. The bleeding does not recur." Ascorbic acid has a known protective action on adrenaline in the circulation.

The electron microscope studies of the capillary bed of ascorbic acid-deficient guinea pigs, by Gore and coworkers (10), published in 1968, disclosed the ultrastructural basis for the capillary defects, the microdiscontinuities and microlesions which lead to capillary fragility.

The above review of the highly suggestive research over the past three decades illustrates the possible usefulness of ascorbic acid in the prevention and treatment of traumatic, hemorrhagic, and surgical shock. Yet how much use is being made of this data in present-day shock therapy? In a paper published in 1969 by Weil and Shubin (11), workers in the Shock Research Unit of a large medical school and hospital, there is not a single mention of ascorbic acid.

With shock still claiming so many victims in highway accidents and battlefield casualties, the need for more work in this area is urgent.

28

PREGNANCY

Pregnancy, parturition, and lactation are periods of intense biochemical stress for mammals. Pregnant mammals, such as rats, which have the ability to produce their own ascorbic acid, significantly increase production of this metabolite to combat these stresses. The recommended daily dietary allowance of ascorbic acid for pregnant and lactating women as set forth by the Food and Nutrition Board of National Academy of Sciences, is 60 milligrams a day (1). Their corresponding recommendations for nonpregnant females, aged eighteen to over seventy-five, is 55 milligrams a day. This provides a meager 5 milligrams a day to maintain homeostasis under the biochemical stresses of a developing baby, the labor of childbirth, the production of milk, and the physiological recovery from the rigors of motherhood itself.

Let us make a simple calculation, assuming that a lactating mother produces 500 to 1,000 milliliters of breast milk daily (about a pint to a quart). This is the amount a normal infant should consume in the first three months of life according to Ingalls (1).

The milk should contain more than 4 milligrams of ascorbic acid per 100 milliliters, according to Snelling (1). This adds up to an additional burden on the mother of 20 to 40 milligrams of ascorbic acid a day which is secreted for the nourishment of the baby. If the lactating mother is only getting a total of 60 milligrams of ascorbic acid a day, this extra load leaves her only 20 to 40 milligrams of ascorbic acid daily for her own hard-working physiology—15 to 35 milligrams a day less than is recommended for a nonlactating female. Draw your own conclusions.

That ascorbic acid is of vital importance in the biochemistry of pregnancy and fetal development can be seen from the profound effects on animals deprived of ascorbic acid. As far back as 1915, before the discovery of ascorbic acid, it was known that the stresses of pregnancy made guinea pigs more susceptible to scurvy. When pregnant guinea pigs were placed on a scorbutic diet early in pregnancy, it led to abortion or absorption of the fetuses, while ascorbic acid deprivation in the latter half of pregnancy resulted in stillbirths or delivery of premature or weak, scorbutic young. Female guinea pigs on a scorbutic diet did not become pregnant and there were profound changes in their ovaries, as described by Kramer and coworkers in 1933. If fed inadequate levels of orange juice, pregnant guinea pigs either aborted or resorbed the fetuses or failed to give birth to living young, depending upon when the experimental animals were deprived of ascorbic acid and the extent of deprivation. Previously, in 1930, it had been shown by Goettsch that depriving guinea pigs of vitamin C not only interfered with the estrus cycle of the females, but the males lost their ability to sire litters. In her paper, Goettsch quoted earlier work, going back to 1919, which showed the deleterious effect of scurvy on the sexual activity of guinea pigs (2).

It is interesting to note in this connection that a simple test, proposed in 1968 by Paeschke and Vasterling (3) to determine the time of ovulation, is based on variations of ascorbic acid in the urine. A marked decrease in urinary ascorbic acid signals the time of ovulation. A similar test was proposed as far back as 1940 by Pillay. Ascorbic acid is also important in the ripening of the human egg, as shown by the 1963 studies of Bertetti and Nonnis-Marzano. This paper contains a bibliography with eighty-five references (3).

As cited in the 1958 paper of Räihä, in a study of over 2,000 women, Martin found an increased frequency of premature births in mothers with the lowest intake levels and lowest serum concentrations of ascorbic acid. In over 200,000 deliveries in Finland, the frequency of stillbirths was highest in December and January and lowest in September. Dietary intakes of ascorbic acid are generally higher in the summer and early fall when fresh fruits and vegetables are available, and they are lowest in the winter months. Pankamaa and Räihä, in 1957, showed a negative correlation between the monthly fluctuations of stillbirths and the ascorbic acid in fetal tissues. Räihä also cited the 1955 paper by Sauvage Nolting, who reported on defective brain development in human subjects caused by ascorbic acid deficiency (4).

In general, it appears that the mother herself suffers more from a diet low in ascorbic acid than the fetus. There seems to be a selective transfer of ascorbic acid by the placenta from the mother's blood to the fetus, as observed by McDevitt in 1942 (5). The ascorbic acid content of the blood of the fetus at birth is higher than the mother's (Manahan and Eastman, 1938; Mindlin, 1940; and Slobody et al., 1946) and the fetus seems to act parasitically (Teel 1938) tending to deplete the mother's supply when her intakes are low. In spite of this, the fetus still may not obtain enough ascorbic acid and congenital scurvy can occur, as shown by Jackson and Park in 1935 (5) and Ingier (2) in 1915.

There is a considerable body of medical literature from 1937 to 1964 indicating that ascorbic acid deficiencies and deprivation are intimately involved with spontaneous abortion, habitual abortion, and premature rupture of the fetal membranes. Therapy which included the use of ascorbic acid proved effective in correcting these conditions (6).

Mammals that produce their own ascorbic acid may not always produce enough to completely overcome the stresses of reproduction and can benefit from additional amounts. It has been reported by Phillips et al. (7), in 1941, that injections of ascorbic acid in "hard to settle" cows resulted in 60 percent of them becoming pregnant on breeding. Similarly, ascorbic acid injections improved the condition of a large percentage of sterile and partially sterile bulls.

Thus, there seems to be general agreement that ascorbic acid deficiency, due to low intakes by the mother during pregnancy, can have serious consequences in the reproductive process. It was only when laboratory animal tests were conducted to determine the effect of added ascorbic acid that contradictory results were obtained which will require further clarification. A program of long-term definitive research work is needed to determine the optimal level of intake for pregnancy, for easing the stresses of parturition and labor, and for the postnatal care of the mother and child.

The following is a brief review of the contradictory data from tests on guinea pigs. In the 1962 publication of the National Research Council of the National Academy of Sciences, "Nutrient Requirements of Laboratory Animals," two diets are given as satisfactory for raising guinea pigs, and hundreds of generations of guinea pigs have probably been raised using them. One diet supplies 12.5 milligrams of ascorbic acid per day, while the other supplies 50 milligrams of ascorbic acid daily. Assuming the guinea pig weighs about 300 grams, these amounts are equivalent to 2.9 grams and 11.7 grams of ascorbic acid respectively for a 70-kilogram body weight (154 pounds).

In 1951, a paper by W. Neuweiler (8) appeared that reported on tests with pregnant guinea pigs which were given 25 milligrams of ascorbic acid daily in addition to their vegetable diet. He stated that, in spite of the fact that there were no general toxic manifestations, there were disturbances to the reproductive process, with fertility changes and increased fetal mortality. He did not mention the number of guinea pigs used in his tests. In 1953, Mouriquand and Edel (8) reported using 250 milligrams of ascorbic acid daily by injection or ingestion (ten times more than Neuweiler used and equivalent to 117 grams of ascorbic acid on a 70-kilogram body weight basis). Males and nonpregnant female guinea pigs were unaffected, but for 3 pregnant females there were shortened gestation periods with increased stillbirths. On the other hand, Lamden and Schweiker (9), in 1955, gave daily intraperitoneal injections of 100 to 200 milligrams of ascorbic acid for six weeks (about 23 grams to 47 grams of ascorbic acid daily for a 70-kilogram body weight) and reported, "There was no interference in the gestation and bearing of healthy litters by two guinea pigs injected with the above amounts of ascorbic acid for a major part of the gestation period."

M. L. Steel (9), in 1968, in a Ph.D. thesis entitled "Growth and Reproduction of Guinea Pigs Fed Three Levels of Ascorbic Acid," used in her work 4, 10, and 100 milligrams per kilogram of body weight (equivalent respectively to 280 milligrams, 700 milligrams, and 7.0 grams per 70-kilogram adult body weight). She showed that animals on the lowest level of ascorbic acid intake had more difficulty in starting a pregnancy, the pregnancy was more likely to end unsuccessfully, the abortion rate was higher, and the death rate was higher. The highest level of ascorbic acid appeared to protect the parent animal from obvious malfunction of the reproductive faculty. However, the survival rate of the offspring was highest when the parent animal was fed the lowest level.

This latter result requires further investigation because it contradicts the results reported in 1967 by C. G. King (9), who supplemented the diet of female guinea pigs each day with 1.5, 3, 6, and 20 milligrams of ascorbic acid. Growth rates were comparable in all groups, but the number of viable offspring increased with each increase in dosage. Survival records were the lowest and stillbirths and resorptions were the highest for the group receiving the least ascorbic acid.

The Soviet worker E. P. Samborskaia (10,, in 1962, tested the effect of ascorbic acid on the reproductive system of guinea pigs and mice and reported changes in the organs and sexual cycles of the animals. According to Steel (9), Samborskaia introduced the ascorbic acid intravaginally into the animals by means of cotton-wool tampons soaked in an ascorbic acid solution, a highly unusual means of application.

In 1964, Samborskaia reported on tests on pregnant guinea pigs given 50 to 500 milligrams of ascorbic acid each day (about 12 to 120 grams per 70 kilograms of body weight), stating that there were increases in abortions, stillbirths, and births of nonviable young. In her 1966 paper, she reported the administration of 150 milligrams of ascorbic acid daily (about 35 grams per 70 kilograms of body weight) to 14 pregnant rats. Three of these rats aborted on the thirteenth to fifteenth day of pregnancy. She also reports tests on women which translate as follows:

> There were twenty women, ages twenty to forty, who had come to the gynecologist with the request for an abortion. Sixteen of the twenty women under observation began to menstruate one to three days after receiving the prescribed course of ascorbic acid. There was no effect on four of the women.

The "prescribed course" appears to have been 6 grams of ascorbic every twenty-four hours for a three-day period. She concluded that this increases the levels of estrogens, which in turn serves to provoke abortion. Besides language difficulties, many Soviet medical papers have a frustrating lack of essential details, but if her results are reliable, then there are wide implications for the use of ascorbic acid in this field, especially since the legalization of abortions. However, many other workers have used ascorbic acid for just the opposite purpose in the treatment of threatened abortion and habitual abortion: Pearse and Trisler (10), in 1957; Ainslee (10), in 1959; and also the numerous workers reporting in the papers cited under reference (6). It is difficult to reconcile the views of this one Soviet worker with the results reported by others.

Samborskaia's work on abortion seems particularly suspicious when viewed in the light of Klenner's results (11), reported in 1971, on megascorbic prophylaxis in over 300 human pregnancies. His patients were given orally, throughout their pregnancies, from 4 grams to 15 grams of ascorbic acid a day on approximately the following schedule: 4 grams daily in the first trimester, 6 grams daily in the second trimester, and 10 grams daily during the last trimester. Approximately 20 percent in this series required 15 grams ascorbic acid a day in the last trimester. There were no miscarriages in the entire series, and one woman in the series had ten consecutive normal pregnancies and ten healthy babies. On admission to the hospital for childbirth, 80 percent of the patients were given a booster injection of 10 grams of ascorbic acid intravenously. Labor was shorter, less painful, and uncomplicated. Striae gravidarum (abdominal wrinkles after childbirth) was seldom seen and there were no postpartum hemorrhages. During childbirth, the perineum was remarkably elastic and episiotomy was performed electively. Healing was always by first intention. Fifteen to twenty years after the last childbirth, the firmness of the perineum is found to be like that during the first childbirth, provided the patient continued on large daily intakes of ascorbic acid. No toxic manifestations were demonstrated in this series and there was no cardiac stress even though twenty-two patients in the series had "rheumatic hearts."

The most remarkable effects of the megascorbic dosages were the health and vigor of the babies. They were all robust and not one required resuscitative measures. All the babies from the series were so strong, good looking, vigorous, and trouble-free that the nurses in the hospital referred to them as the "Vitamin C Babies." The Fultz quadruplets were in this series and they are the only quadruplets that have survived in southeastern United States. The babies were given 50 milligrams of ascorbic acid on the first day and dose was gradually increased thereafter until they were taking 1 gram a day at one year of age. This recommended routine daily dose is increased 1 gram for each year of age until ten years and then 10 grams regularly thereafter. This megascorbic regimen in pregnancy and childbirth certainly deserves wider recognition and use.

For the induction of labor in childbirth, the administration of ascorbic acid was proposed by Spitzer (12), in 1947; and Tasch (12), in 1951, used it to shorten the period of labor and to favorably influence the postlabor period. McCormick (12), in 1948, suggested ascorbic acid as a means of avoiding the striae of pregnancy (striae gravidarum or striae atrophicae). Further research would also be profitable in these areas and also in the treatment of painful menstruation (13), excessive menstrual bleeding (14), and in relief of menopausal disorders (15).

29

MENTAL DISEASES

One area where considerable research with ascorbic acid has been expended is in the treatment of schizophrenia. A substantial amount of clinical information has been collected in the chemotherapy of this disease using the megascorbic and megavitamin approach. In a 1967 report (1) of twelve independent psychiatric studies, 80 percent of 1,500 schizophrenics, continuously treated with megascorbic and megavitamin therapy, showed recovery or marked improvement. It was estimated that 1,500 doctors in the United States and Canada and over a hundred institutions were using this treatment.

At the present time this research and therapy are continuing at a rapid pace and a publicly supported foundation, the American Schizophrenia Foundation, not only has been involved in much of this research, but also has plans for organizing a research and demonstration facility, which will eventually carry a patient load of 3,000 to 5,000 annually. Biochemical investigations of mental diseases will be conducted in this facility which will also act as a training facility for doctors. Further information is available from this foundation and from its chapters in many states, Canada, and Bolivia.

In 1884, J. W. L. Thudichum (2), who is regarded by many as the father of modern neurochemistry, published a book on brain chemistry in which he advanced the hypothesis that "many forms of insanity" are caused by "poisons fermented within the body," that is, toxic substances produced or delivered to the brain by a faulty metabolism. He also suggested that these unknown processes would become quite obvious when we acquired a better understanding of the biochemistry of the brain. He spent the next ten years in the isolation and characterization of some of the chemical constituents of the brain. However, it is only the research of the past several decades that has confirmed his keen foresight.

The discovery and synthesis of ascorbic acid initiated such a large volume of research that, in 1938, Wacholder compiled a review to determine the extent of the interest of this work for neurology and psychiatry. In 1940, Lucksch reported his results in his paper, "Vitamin C and Schizophrenia." Also in 1940, Soloveva, from the Soviet Union, reported favorable results from its use in various psychoses. Berkenau, in 1940, suggested that the delay in the ascorbic acid "saturation" of his small group of psychotic patients may be significant. In 1951, another review by Low-Maus, 'Vitamin C and the Nervous System," appeared with seventy-six references (3).

In the period from 1953 to 1955, De Sauvage Nolting (4) published a series of short papers on the relation of ascorbic acid to mental disease. From 1957 to 1966, there appeared papers published in various parts of the world which showed that mental disease patients have high demands for ascorbic acid, have subnormal body levels, and, in many cases, are in a state of subclinical scurvy. Several of the papers suggested that mental patients should be given large doses of ascorbic acid (5).

VanderKamp (6), in 1966, found that schizophrenics metabolized ascorbic acid at a rate 10 times that of a control group. He gave 6 to 8 grams of ascorbic acid every 4 hours to a group of ten schizophrenics, or a total of 36 to 48 grams of ascorbic acid a day. All ten of the patients showed definite clinical improvement.

This review indicates the practical usefulness of massive doses of ascorbic acid in the treatment of schizophrenia, but it does not give us much information as to how it works or any insight as to what are Thudichum's "poisons fermented within the body" which may cause mental illness.

In the case of schizophrenia, a brilliant series of research papers, started in the early 1950s by A. Hoffer, H. Osmond, and their coworkers (7), has brought much light into this area and has been a major factor in confirming Thudichum's insight. It has also served to return the biochemistry of the body to psychiatry after a long attempt to exile it in favor of culture and psyche. This research was based on a hypothesis which resulted from two simple observations (8):

1. There is a chemical similarity between adrenalin, the normal secretion of the adrenal gland, and mescaline, a hallucinatory drug.
2. The psychological effects of mescaline on humans in many ways resemble the symptoms of acute schizophrenia. The faulty metabolism of adrenalin in the body of a schizophrenic, possibly due to a genetic defect (9), could lead to an adrenalin metabolite with psychological properties resembling those of mescaline, but much more potent. If such a substance were made in the body, then clinical schizophrenia would result.

It was suggested that the faulty metabolism of adrenalin led to an increased production of adrenochrome, which they showed was an hallucinogen. Their hypothesis suggested that the adrenochrome was partially responsible for the changes produced in schizophrenia, and it would follow that any method for decreasing adrenochrome production from adrenalin would be therapeutic for schizophrenia. This was attempted by using massive doses of the vitamin, niacin, to reduce the formation of the precursor, adrenalin, from noradrenalin. Clinical experience has been good and has shown the value of including high levels of the other B vitamins in the therapy. Ascorbic acid is also used at levels of 1 to 6 grams a day and the reasons for using ascorbic acid were the subject of a comprehensive paper by Hoffer and Osmond (5). Their research has been long and continuing and its reception has been stormy, which is the usual course for a new concept. The final test is in the clinical results, which appear good.

Linus Pauling (10), in a 1967 paper entitled, "Orthomolecular Somatic and Psychiatric Medicine," proposed a new means of treating disease. The therapy merely provides the optimal molecular constitution of the body, especially the optimal concentration of substances which are normally present in the human body and are required for life itself. It is known that the proper functioning of the mind requires the presence in the brain of molecules of many different substances, such as the B vitamins and ascorbic acid, and malfunction may result if optimal levels are not maintained. This work, which provides the rationale for the use of large doses of normal metabolites in the treatment of mental disease, was further elaborated in a paper on "Orthomolecular Psychiatry" in 1968. In a talk presented at the Second International Conference of Social Psychiatry in London in 1969, Pauling suggested that an optimal intake of ascorbic acid could mean a 10 percent improvement in physical and mental health. He speculated, "What would be the consequences for the world if the national leaders and the people as a whole were to think just 10 percent more clearly?"

The effect of continued mega levels of ascorbic acid on human intelligence is a subject which has never been examined. Tests could easily be applied on two populations of children from similar backgrounds and economic levels. One group would be maintained on their present intake levels of ascorbic acid from their foodstuffs, which inadequately corrects their hypoascorbemia, and the other group continuously maintained (from birth, if possible) on the levels, suggested by Dr. F. R. Klenner, of 1 gram ascorbic acid per day, per year of age, up to age of ten, and then 10 grams a day thereafter. Some startling improvements on intelligence levels may be observed by this orthomolecular approach.

As in other chapters, this review must be brief and incomplete. Because of limited space, many important references containing significant contributions to this work have been omitted. If the reader is interested, reference may be made to a recent more detailed review (11) which cites 191 references.

Happily, in the concluding chapter, some organized research can be cited in megascorbic and megavitamin therapy which has yielded definite benefits. It is hoped that this is only the beginning of a trend in organized and coordinated research in megascorbic therapy.

30

THE FUTURE

The large amount of medical literature cited in Chapters 12 to 29 represents but a small fraction of the total work published during the last forty years on the use of ascorbic acid for diseases other than scurvy. This vast volume of research time and energy was expended by hundreds of workers scattered all over the world with a complete lack of coordination of their experimental techniques, purpose, and background. Their total effort has settled few problems of practical importance and has resulted, at best, in many suggestions for future research. The bulk of this uncoordinated effort has produced a gigantic waste of time and money and a confusing mass of conflicting results and opinions. While these four decades of work have established the dosage of ascorbic acid necessary to prevent frank clinical scurvy, we still are not sure of such simple facts as the optimal intakes of ascorbic acid needed for good health and resistance to disease processes, and how dosage requirements vary from individual to individual and under stress. Past research, because of its haphazard nature, lack of coordinated effort, and inability to carry an investigation to its ultimate final solution, has created more problems than it has solved. Much greater progress should have been made in these last forty years than has actually occurred.

To avoid these pitfalls in future research, and because of the broad range of potential uses of ascorbic acid, the establishment of a central agency, to coordinate, initiate, sponsor, and direct the future research effort is required. Such an agency would also act as a clearinghouse for pertinent information and regularly publish, at frequent intervals, the results of the current research. Most important is the staffing of that agency. It should be a multidisciplinary group of unbiased, imaginative scientists with a wide background on the modern concepts of ascorbic acid; it should comprise clinicians, M.D.'s, biochemists, and scientists from other disciplines to tackle every possible problem.

The National Institutes of Health in Bethesda, Maryland, could set up and organize a new division, "Hyposascorbemia and Mega-ascorbic Medicine," to function in this capacity. If Congress could be convinced of the urgent need for this concentrated effort and its probable beneficial effects on American public health, it could direct the Department of Health, Education, and Welfare to accomplish this. It is the fond hope of the author that, as further research is conducted on hypoascorbemia and the realization of its importance is confirmed, a National Megascorbic Authority will eventually be organized with general aims and purposes similar to the proposed National Cancer Authority.

No claim is made for the complete coverage of the subject matter of Chapters 12 to 29. Other areas of investigation would be part of the program of the agency, such as verifying the reports of the beneficial action of ascorbic acid in multiple sclerosis, Meniere's syndrome, hemophilia, and insomnia, to name a few. The megavitamin therapy of schizophrenia is now actively being investigated by the publicly supported American Schizophrenia Association and the Huxley Institute for Biosocial Research. These new agencies could cooperate and work closely with these foundations.

The main purpose of this agency would be to determine the optimal levels of ascorbic acid intakes based on the genetic concepts, under "normal" and stressed conditions, and the human individual variations and responses. Such an agency could determine the safety of megascorbic prophylaxis and megascorbic therapy, and make available practical applications of these measures with the shortest time lag. Presently, we can only entertain a hope that future generations may live longer and healthier lives because of these ideas.

Another factor which has impeded the development of the wider usage of ascorbic acid in megascorbic prophylaxis and megascorbic therapy has been a lack of convenient dosage forms for these purposes. For oral administration, the largest easily available tablet contains only 500 milligrams and the largest chewable tablet has 250 milligrams of ascorbic acid. If one wants to consume 10 grams of ascorbic acid a day, it is necessary to swallow twenty large tablets or eat forty chewables. The less readily available powdered ascorbic acid or sodium ascorbate, when measured by the teaspoonful (a level teaspoonful is about 3 grams) and dissolved in water or fruit juice, is convenient and palatable when obtainable. This also avoids the possibility of discomfort when swallowing a series of large tablets. What is really needed for oral administration is a pleasantly flavored chewable wafer supplying 2 or 3 grams of ascorbic acid.

The situation is even worse for doctors who want to use mega-ascorbic therapy by injection. The only injectable ascorbic acid now available in the trade comes in small ampuls containing, at most, 1 gram of ascorbic acid. If a doctor wants to administer a therapeutic injection of 30 or 40 grams, he must break open and combine the contents of at least thirty or forty small glass ampuls in order to obtain the required dosage. Only an unusually dedicated physician will go to this trouble. What is needed here is a wide distribution of large ampuls with sterile solutions containing 20 to 40 grams of sodium ascorbate suitable for injection. Similarly, for longer-term parenteral fluid therapy by the intravenous route, bottles of parenteral solutions containing up to 30 grams of sodium ascorbate per liter are needed. The only product distributed at present is a vitamin mixture containing, at most, about a gram of vitamin C per liter. The availability of these products would make megascorbic therapy, for the practicing physician in his office and hospital, a practical reality for both emergencies and routine therapy.

REFERENCES CITED FROM THE MEDICAL LITERATURE

Chapter 12 — The Common Cold

1. C. W. Jungeblut. A Further Contribution to the Vitamin C Therapy in Experimental Poliomyelitis. *Journal of Experimental Medicine,* vol. 70: p. 327. 1939.

2. G. Berquist. *Svenska läktidning,* vol. 37: pp. 1149-1158. 1940.

3. A. G. Kuttner. Effect of Large Doses of Vitamins A, B, C and D on the Incidence of Upper Respiratory Infections in a Group of Rheumatic Children. *Journal Clinical Investigation,* vol. 19: pp. 809–812. 1940.

4. D. W. Cowan et al. Vitamins for the Prevention of Colds. *Journal American Medical Association,* vol. 120: pp. 1268–1271. 1942.

5 A. J. Glazebrook and S. Thomson. The Administration of Vitamin C in a Large Institution and Its Effect on General

Health and Resistance to Infection. *Journal of Hygiene,* vol. 12: pp. 1–19. 1942.

6. G. Dahlberg et al. Ascorbic Acid as a Prophylactic Agent Against Common Colds. *Acta Medica Scandinavica,* vol. 119: pp. 540–561. 1944.

7. W. Franz and H. L. Heyl. Blood Levels of Ascorbic Acid in Bioflavonoid and Ascorbic Acid Therapy of the Common Cold. *Journal American Medical Association,* vol. 162: pp. 1224–1226. 1956.

8. H. E. Tebrock et al. Usefulness of Bioflavonoids and Ascorbic Acid in Treatment of Common Cold. *Journal American Medical Association,* vol. 162: pp. 1227–1233. 1956.

9. G. A. Shekhtman. On the Significance of Continuous Addition of Vitamin C to Food in a Military Sector. *Voenno-Meditsinskii Zhurnal* (Moskva), vol. 3: pp. 46–49, 1961.

10. S. L. Ruskin. Calcium Cevitamate (Calcium Ascorbate) in the Treatment of Acute Rhinitis. *Annals Otology, Rhinology and Laryngology,* vol. 47: pp. 502–511. 1938.

11. O. E. Van Alyea. The Acute Nasal Infection. *Nebraska State Medical Journal,* vol. 27: pp. 265–274. 1942.

12. N. W. Markwell. Vitamin C in the Prevention of Colds. *Medical Journal of Australia,* vol. 34: pp. 777–778. 1947.

13. P. Albanese. Treatment of Respiratory Infections with High Doses of Vitamin C. *El Dia Medico,* vol. 19: pp. 1738–1740. 1947.

14. A. S. Woolstone. Treatment of the Common Cold. *British Medical Journal,* vol. 2: p. 1290. 1954.

15. H. Miegl. Acute Infections of the Upper Respiratory Tract and Their Treatment with Vitamin C. *Wiener Medizinische Wochenschrift,* vol. 107: pp. 989–992, 1957. The Use of Vitamin C in Otorhinolaryngology. Ibid., vol. 108: pp. 859–864. 1958.

16. C. Bessel-Lorch. Common Cold Prophylaxis in Young People at a Ski Camp. *Medizinische Welt,* vol. 44: pp. 2126–2127. 1959.

17. G. Ritzel. Critical Evaluation of Vitamin C as a Prophylactic and Therapeutic Agent in Colds. *Helvetia Medica Acta,* vol. 2: pp. 63–68. 1961.

18. L. Pauling. *Vitamin C and the Common Cold.* San Francisco, California: W. H. Freeman and Company. 1970.

Chapter 13 — Viral Infection

1. C. W. Jungeblut. Inactivation of Poliomyelitis Virus by Crystalline Vitamin C (Ascorbic Acid). *Journal of Experimental Medicine,* vol. 62: pp. 517–521. 1935.

2. M. Holden and R. J. Resnick. In Vitro Action of Synthetic Crystalline Vitamin C (Ascorbic Acid) on Herpes Virus. *Journal of Immunology,* vol. 31: pp. 455–462. 1936.

   M. Holden and E. Molloy. Further Experiments on Inactivation of Herpes Virus by Vitamin C (1-ascorbic acid). Ibid., vol. 33: pp. 251–257. 1937.

3. I. J. Kligler and H. Bernkopf. Inactivation of Vaccinia Virus by Ascorbic Acid and Glutathione. *Nature,* vol. 139: pp. 965–966. 1937.

4. W. Langenbusch and A. Enderling. Einfluss der Vitamine auf das Virus der Maul-und Klavenseuch. *Zentralblatt fur Bakteriologie,* vol. 140: pp. 112–115. 1937.

5. G. Amato. Azione dell'acido ascorbico sul virus fisso della rabbia e sulla tossina tetanica. *Giornale di Batteriologia, Virologia et Immunologia* (Torino), vol. 19: pp. 843–849. 1937.

6. I. Lominski. Inactivation du bacteriophage par l'acide ascorbique. *Comptes Rendus des Séances de la Société de Biologie et de Ses Filiales* (Paris), vol. 122: pp. 766–768. 1936.

7. M. Lojkin. *Contributions of the Boyce Thompson Institute,* vol. 8, No. 4. 1936. L. F. Martin. Proceedings Third International Congress of Microbiology, New York, 1940, p. 281.

8. C. W. Jungeblut. Further Observations on Vitamin C

Therapy in Experimental Poliomyelitis. *Journal of Experimental Medicine,* vol. 65: pp. 127–146. 1937. Ibid., vol. 66: pp. 459–477, 1937. Ibid., vol. 70: pp. 315–332. 1939.

9. A. B. Sabin. Vitamin C in Relation to Experimental Poliomyelitis, *Journal of Experimental Medicine,* vol. 69: pp. 507–515. 1939.

10. F. R. Klenner. The Treatment of Poliomyelitis and Other Virus Diseases with Vitamin C. *Southern Medicine and Surgery,* vol. 111: pp. 209–214. 1949. Massive Doses of Vitamin C and the Virus Diseases. Ibid., vol. 113: pp. 101–107. 1951. The Vitamin and Massage Treatment for Acute Poliomyelitis. Ibid., vol. 114: pp. 194–197. 1952. The Use of Vitamin C as an Antibiotic. *Journal of Applied Nutrition,* vol. 6: pp. 274–278. 1953. The Folly in the Continued Use of a Killed Polio Virus Vaccine. *Tri-State Medical Journal,* pp. 1–8. Feb. 1959.

11. O. Gsell and F. Kalt. Treatment of Epidemic Poliomyelitis with High Doses of Ascorbic Acid. *Schweizerische Medizinische Wochenschrift,* vol. 84: pp. 661-666. 1954.

12. H. Baur. Poliomyelitis Therapy with Ascorbic Acid. *Helvetia Medica Acta,* vol. 19: pp. 470–474. 1952.

13. E. Greer. Vitamin C in Acute Poliomyelitis. *Medical Times* (Manhasset), vol. 83: pp. 1160–1161. 1955.

14. O. A. Bessey et al. Pathologic Changes in Organs of Scorbutic Guinea Pigs. *Proceedings Society Experimental Biology and Medicine,* vol. 31: pp. 455–460. 1934.

15. W. O. Russell and C. P. Calloway. Pathologic Changes in the Liver and Kidneys of Guinea Pigs Deficient in Vitamin C. *Archives of Pathology,* vol. 35: pp. 546–552. 1943.

16. G. C. Willis. The Influence of Ascorbic Acid upon the Liver. *Canadian Medical Association Journal,* vol. 76: pp. 1044–1048. 1957.

17. H. Baur and H. Staub. Therapy of Hepatitis with Ascorbic Acid Infusions. *Schweizerische Medizinische Wochenschrift,* vol. 84: pp. 595–597. 1954.

18. F. Spengler. Vitamin C und der Diuretische Effekt bei Le-

berzirrhose. *München Medizinische Wochenschrift*, vol. 84: pp. 779–780. 1937.

19. H. Kirchmair. Treatment of Epidemic Hepatitis in Children with High Doses of Ascorbic Acid. *Medizinische Monatschrift*, vol. 11: pp. 353–357. 1957. Ascorbic Acid Treatment of Epidemic Hepatitis in Children. *Deutsche Gesundheitwesen*, vol. 12: pp. 773–774. 1957. Epidemic Hepatitis in Children and Its Treatment with High Doses of Ascorbic Acid. Ibid., vol. 12: pp. 1525–1536. 1957.

20. H. B. Calleja and R. H. Brooks. Acute Hepatitis Treated with High Doses of Vitamin C. *Ohio State Medical Journal*, vol. 56: pp. 821–823. 1960.

21. D. Baetgen. Results of the Treatment of Epidemic Hepatitis in Children with High Doses of Ascorbic Acid in the Years 1957–1958. *Medizinische Monatschrift*, vol. 15: pp. 30–36. 1961.

22. W. L. Dalton. Massive Doses of Vitamin C in the Treatment of Viral Diseases. *Journal Indiana State Medical Association*, vol. 55: pp. 1151–1154. 1962.

23. I. Dainow. Treatment of Herpes Zoster with Vitamin C. *Dermatologia*, vol. 68: pp. 197–201. 1943.

24. M. Zureick. Treatment of Shingles and Herpes with Vitamin C Intravenously. *Journal des Praticiens*, vol. 64: p. 586. 1950.

25. F. R. Klenner. Virus Pneumonia and Its Treatment with Vitamin C. *Southern Medicine and Surgery*, vol. 110: pp. 36–46. 1948.

26. J. M. Paez de la Torre. Ascorbic Acid in Measles. *Archives Argentinos de Pediatria*, vol. 24: pp. 225–227. 1945.

27. R. Vargas Magne. Vitamin C in Treatment of Influenza. *El Dia Medico*, vol. 35: pp. 1714-1715. 1963.

28. J. B. Enright. Geographical Distribution of Bat Rabies in the United States, 1953–1960. *American Journal of Public Health*, vol. 52: pp. 484–488. 1962.

29. G. L. Humphrey et al. Fatal Case of Rabies in a Woman

Bitten by a Bat. *Public Health Reports,* vol. 75: pp. 317–326, 1960. J. R. Kent. Human Rabies Transmitted by the Bite of a Bat. *New England Journal of Medicine,* vol. 263: pp. 1058–1065. 1960.

Chapter 14 — Bacterial Infection

1. G. C. D. Gupta and B. C. Guha. The Effect of Vitamin C and Certain Other Substances on the Growth of Microorganisms. *Annals Biochemistry and Experimental Medicine,* vol. 1: pp. 14–26. 1941.

2. C. H. Boissevain and J. H. Spillane. Effect of Ascorbic Acid on Growth of Tuberculosis Bacillus. *American Review of Tuberculosis,* vol. 35: pp. 661–662. 1937.

3. M. Sirsi. Antimicrobial Action of Vitamin C on M. Tuberculosis and Some Other Pathogenic Organisms. *Indian Journal of Medical Sciences* (Bombay), vol. 6: pp. 252–255. 1952.

4. Q. Myrvik et al. Studies on the Tuberculoinhibitory Properties of Ascorbic Acid Derivatives and Their Possible Role in Inhibition of Tubercle Bacilli by Urine. *American Review of Tuberculosis,* vol. 69: pp. 406–418. 1954.

5. E. Harde and M. M. Phillippe. Observations on the Antigenic Activities of Combined Diphtheria Toxin and Vitamin C. *Comptes Rendus Hebdomadaires des Séances de l'Academie des Sciences,* vol. 199: pp. 738–739. 1934.
   C. L. Jungeblut and R. L. Zwemer. Inactivation of Diphtheria Toxin in Vivo and in Vitro by Crystalline Vitamin C (Ascorbic Acid). *Proceedings Society of Experimental Biology and Medicine,* vol. 32: pp. 1229-1234. 1935.
   A. Sigal and C. G. King. The Influence of Vitamin C Deficiency upon the Resistance of Guinea Pigs to Diphtheria Toxin. *Journal of Pharmacology and Experimental Therapeutics,* vol. 61: pp. 1–9. 1937.
   I. J. Kligler et al. Effect of Ascorbic Acid on Toxin Production of C. Diphtheriae in Culture Media. *Journal of Pathology and Bacteriology* (London), vol. 45: pp. 414–429. 1937.

6. C. W. Jungeblut. Inactivation of Tetanus Toxin by

Crystalline Vitamin C (Ascorbic Acid). *Journal of Immunol ogy,* vol. 33: pp. 203–214. 1937.

I. J. Kligler et al. Influence of Ascorbic Acid on the Growth and Toxin Production of C1. tetani and on the Detoxication of Tetanus Toxin. *Journal of Pathology and Bacteriology* (London), vol. 46: pp. 619–629. 1938.

E. Schulze and V. Hecht. Uber die Wirkung der Ascorbin-saure zur Diphtherie-Formol-Toxoid und Tetanus Toxin. *Klinische Wochenschrift,* vol. 16: pp. 1460–1463. 1937.

K. Kuribayashi et al. Effect of Vitamin C on Bacterial Toxins. *Japanese Journal of Bacteriology,* vol. 18: pp. 136–142. 1963.

7. T. Kodama and T. Kojima. Studies of the Staphylococcal Toxin, Toxoid and Antitoxin; Effect of Ascorbic Acid on Staphylococcal Lysins and Organisms. *Kitasato Archives of Experimental Medicine,* vol. 16: pp. 36–55. 1939.

8. Z. Takahashi. *Nagoya Journal of Medical Science,* vol. 12: p. 50. 1938.

E. Cottingham and C. A. Mills. Influence of Temperature and Vitamin Deficiency upon Phagocytic Functions. *Journal of Immunology,* vol. 47: pp. 493–502. 1943.

L. R. DeChatelet et al. Ascorbic Acid: Possible Role in Phagocytosis. Paper read at 62nd Meeting, American Society of Biological Chemists, San Francisco, June 18, 1971.

M. R. Cooper et al. Stimulation of Leukocyte Hexose Mono-phosphate Shunt Activity by Ascorbic Acid. *Infection and Immunity,* vol. 3: pp. 851–853. 1971.

9. J. M. Faulkner and F. H. L. Taylor. Vitamin C and Infection. *Annals of Internal Medicine,* vol. 10: pp. 1867–1873. 1937.

L. J. Harris et al. Influence of Infection on the Vitamin C Content of the Tissues of Animals. *Lancet,* vol. 2: pp. 183–186. 1937.

D. Perla and J. Marmorsten. Role of Vitamin C in Resistance. *Archives of Pathology,* vol. 23: pp. 543–575, 683–712. 1937.

10. M. McConkey and D. T. Smith. The Relation of Vitamin C Deficiency to Intestinal Tuberculosis in the Guinea Pig.

Journal of Experimental Medicine, vol. 58: pp. 503–512. 1933.

11. E. de Savitsch et al. The Influence of Orange Juice on Experimental Tuberculosis in Guinea Pigs. *National Tuberculosis Association Transactions,* vol. 30: pp. 130–135. 1934.

    M. R. Greene et al. Role of Chronic Vitamin C Deficiency in Pathogenesis of Tuberculosis in Guinea Pigs. *American Review of Tuberculosis,* vol. 33: pp. 585–624. 1936.

    K. E. Birkhaug. The Role of Vitamin C in the Pathogenesis of Tuberculosis in the Guinea Pig. I to V. *Acta Tuberculosis Scandinavica,* vol. 12: pp. 89–98, 98–104, 359–372. 1938. Ibid., vol. 13: pp. 45–51, 52–66. 1939.

12. F. Heise. Supervitaminosis C. *Proceedings Society Experimental Biology and Medicine,* vol. 35: pp. 337–338. 1936. Vitamin C Immunity in Tuberculosis in Guinea Pigs. *American Review of Tuberculosis,* vol. 39: pp. 794–795. 1939.

13. P. Kleimenhagen. Effect of Ascorbic Acid on Experimental Tuberculosis in Guinea Pigs. *Zeitschrift fur Vitaminforschung,* vol. 11: pp. 209–227. 1941.

    M. M. Steinbach and S. J. Klein. Vitamin C in Experimental Tuberculosis. *American Review of Tuberculosis,* vol. 43: pp. 403–414. 1941.

    S. V. Boyden and M. E. Andersen. Diet and Experimental Tuberculosis in the Guinea Pig. *Acta Pathologica et Microbiologica Scandinavica* (Kobenhavn), vol. 39: pp. 107–116. 1956.

14. F. H. Heise and G. J. Martin. Ascorbic Acid Metabolism in Tuberculosis. *Proceedings Society Experimental Biology and Medicine,* vol. 34: pp. 642–644. 1936.

    F. Hasselbach. Vitamin C und Lungentuberkulose. Veraussetzungen Beabachtungen und Erfahrungen bei der Behandlung Lungentuberkuloser. *Zeitschrift fur Tuberkulose und Erkranken der Thoraxovgane* (Leipsig), vol. 75: pp. 336–347. 1936.

    M. A. Abbasy et al. Journal Society Chemical Industry, vol. 55: pp. 841 to end. 1936.

    J. C. Degeller. Acta Brevie Neerland Physiologie, *Pharma-*

cologie et Microbiologie, vol. 6: pp. 64 to end. 1936.

W. W. Jetter and T. S. Bombalo. The Urinary Output of Vitamin C in Active Tuberculosis in Children. *American Journal of Medical Science,* vol. 195: pp. 362–366. 1938.

H. Alexander. Vitamin C and Tuberculosis. *Deutsches Tuberkulose-Blatt,* vol. 14: pp. 125–130. 1940.

M. Pijoan and B. Sedlacek. Ascorbic Acid in Tuberculous Navajo Indians. *American Review of Tuberculosis,* vol. 48: pp. 342–346. 1943.

J. E. Sylvestre and M. Giroux. Vitamin C Therapy of Pulmonary Tuberculosis. *Laval Medical* (Quebec), vol. 10: pp. 417–427. 1945.

15. H. A. Getz et al. A Study of the Relation of Nutrition to the Development of Tuberculosis. *American Review of Tuberculosis,* vol. 64: pp. 381–393. 1951.

16. F. Hasselbach. Therapy of Tuberculosis Pulmonary Hemorrhages with Vitamin C. *Fortschrift der Therapie,* vol. 7: pp. 407–411. 1935.

M. Radford et al. Blood Changes Following Continuous Daily Administration of Vitamin C and Orange Juice to Tuberculous Patients. *American Review of Tuberculosis,* vol. 35: pp. 784 to end. 1937.

G. Borsalino. La Fragilita Capillare Nella Tubercolosi Polmonare e le Sue Modificazioni per Azione Della Vitamin C. *Giornale di Clinica Medica* (Bologna), vol. 18: pp. 273-294. 1937.

G. J. Martin and F. H. Heise. Vitamin C Nutrition on Pulmonary Tuberculosis. *American Journal Digestive Diseases and Nutrition,* vol. 4: pp. 368–373. 1937.

C. K. Petter. Vitamin C and Tuberculosis. *The Journal-Lancet* (Minneapolis), vol. 57: pp. 221–224. 1937.

E. Albrecht. Vitamin C as an Adjuvant in the Therapy of Lung Tuberculosis. *Medizinische Klinik* (München), vol. 34: pp. 972–973. 1938.

A. Josewich. Value of Vitamin C Therapy in Lung Tuberculosis. *Medical Bulletin of the Veterans Administration,* vol. 16: pp. 8–11. 1939.

I. Baksh and M. Rabbani. Vitamin C in Pulmonary Tuberculosis. *Indian Medical Gazette,* vol. 74: pp. 274–277. 1939.

17. G. S. Erwin et al. Hypovitaminosis C and Pulmonary Tuberculosis. *British Medical Journal*, vol. 1: pp. 688–689. 1940.

A. Kaplan and M. E. Zounis. Vitamin C in Pulmonary Tuberculosis. *American Review of Tuberculosis*, vol. 42: pp. 667–673. 1940.

H. C. Sweany et al. The Body Economy of Vitamin C in Health and Disease. *Journal American Medical Association*, vol. 116: pp. 469-474. 1941.

J. R. B. Vitorero and J. Doyle. Treatment of Intestinal Tuberculosis with Vitamin C. *Medical Weekly*, vol. 2: pp. 636–640. 1938.

E. Bogen et al. Vitamin C Treatment of Mucous Membrane Tuberculosis. *American Review of Tuberculosis*, vol. 44: pp. 596–603. 1941.

M. N. Rudra and S. K. Roy. Haematological Study in Pulmonary Tuberculosis and the Effect upon It of Large Doses of Vitamin C. *Tubercle*, vol. 27: pp. 93–94. 1946.

I. J. Babbar. Therapeutic Effect of Ascorbic Acid in Tuberculosis. *Indian Medical Gazette*, vol. 83: pp. 409–410. 1948.

18. J. Charpy. Ascorbic Acid in Very Large Doses Alone or with Vitamin D2 in Tuberculosis. *Bulletin de l'Academie Nationale de Médecine* (Paris), vol. 132: pp. 421–423. 1948.

19. A. Hochwald. Observations on the Effect of Ascorbic Acid on Croupous Pneumonia. *Wien Archiv fur Innere Medizin*, vol. 29: pp. 353–374. 1936.

J. Gander and W. Niederberger. Vitamin C in the Treatment of Pneumonia. *Münchener Medizinische Wochenschrift*, vol. 51: pp. 2074 to end. 1936.

W. Gunzel and G. Kroehnert. Experiences in the Treatment of Pneumonia with Vitamin C. *Fortschrifte der Therapie*, vol. 13: pp. 460–463. 1937.

H. Kienart. Treatment of Croupous Pneumonia With Vitamin C. *Münchener Medizinische Wochenschrift*, vol. 23: pp. 913 to end. 1939.

F. Szirmai. Value of Vitamin C in Treatment of Acute Infectious Diseases. *Deutsches Archive fur Klinische Medizin*, vol. 85: pp. 434-443. 1940.

W. Stein. The Role of Vitamin and Adrenal Cortex Hormone in the Treatment of Pneumococcal Pneumonias. *Medical Bulletin of the Veterans Administration*, vol. 18: pp. 156–160. 1941.

G. Biilmann. Ascorbic Acid Treatment of Croupous Pneumonia. *Acta Medica Scandinavica*, suppl. 123: pp. 102–106. 1941.

D. D. Chacko. A Note on the Use of Vitamin C in Arteriosclerosis. *Journal of the Christian Medical Association of India*, vol. 27: p. 277. 1952.

20. O. Grootten and N. Bezssonoff. Action of Vitamin C on Diphtheria Toxin. *Annales de l'Institute Pasteur*, vol. 56: pp. 413–426. 1936.

T. Otani. On the Vitamin C Therapy of Whooping Cough. *Klinische Wochenschrift*, vol. 15: pp. 1884–1885. 1936. Influence of Vitamin C (1-Ascorbic Acid) upon the Whooping Cough Bacillus and Its Toxin. *Oriental Journal of Diseases of Infants*, vol. 25: pp. 1–4. 1939.

21. M. J. Ormerod, et al. A Further Report on the Ascorbic Acid Treatment of Whooping Cough. *Canadian Medical Association Journal*, vol. 37: pp. 268–272. 1937.

A. Plate. Treatment of Whooping Cough with Vitamin C. *Kinderaerztliche Praxis* (Leipsig), vol. 8: pp. 70–71. 1937.

D. Gairdner. Vitamin C in the Treatment of Whooping Cough. *British Medical Journal*, vol. 2: pp. 742–744. 1938.

E. L. Vermillion and G. E. Stafford. A Preliminary Report on the Use of Cevitamic Acid in the Treatment of Whooping Cough. *Journal of the Kansas Medical Society*, vol. 39: pp. 469 and 479. 1938.

22. T. Sessa. Vitamin Therapy of Whooping Cough. *Riforma Medica*, vol. 56: pp. 38–43. 1940.

K. Meier. Vitamin C Treatment of Pertussis. *Annales de Pédiatrie* (Paris), vol. 164: pp. 50–53. 1945.

23. L. Pfeiffer. Ascorbic Acid Therapy of Whooping Cough. *Helvetica Paediatrica Acta* (Basel), vol. 2: pp. 106–112. 1947.

J. C. DeWit. Treatment of Whooping Cough with Vitamin C. *Kindergeneeskunde*, vol. 17: pp. 367–374. 1949.

24. L. M. Bechelli. Vitamin C Therapy of the Lepra Reaction. *Revista Brasileira de Leprologia* (Sao Paulo), vol. 7: pp. 251–255. 1939.

C. Gatti and R. J. Gaona. Ascorbic Acid in the Treatment of Leprosy. *Archiv Schiffe-und Tropenhygiene,* vol. 43: pp. 32–33. 1939.

R. G. Ugarizza. Ascorbic Acid in the Treatment of Leprous Septicemia. *Archiv Schiffe-und Tropenhygiene,* vol. 43: pp. 33–34. 1939.

D. L. Ferreira. Vitamin C in Leprosy. *Publicacöes Medicas,* vol. 20: pp. 25–28. 1950.

H. Floch and P. Sureau. Vitamin C Therapy in Leprosy. *Bulletin de la Société de Pathologie Exotique et de Ses Filiales* (Paris), vol. 45: pp. 443–446. 1952.

25. N. Farah. Enteric Fever Treated with Suprarenal Cortex Extract and Vitamin C Intravenously. *Lancet,* vol. 1: pp. 777–779. 1938.

J. Drummond. Recent Advances in the Treatment of Enteric Fever. *Clinical Proceedings* (South Africa), vol. 2: pp. 65–93. 1943.

26. E. H. Sadun et al. Effect of Ascorbic Acid Deficiency on the Resistance of Guinea Pigs to Infection with Endamoeba Histolytica of Human Origin. *American Journal of Tropical Medicine,* vol. 31: pp. 426–437. 1951.

T. A. Veselovskaia. Effect of Vitamin C on the Clinical Course of Dysentery. *Voenno-Meditsinskii Zhurnal* (Moskva), No. 3: pp. 32–37. 1957.

V. S. Sokolova. Application of Vitamin C in Treatment of Dysentery. *Terapevticheskii Arkhiv* (Moskva), vol. 30: pp. 59–64. 1958.

27. J. Dujardin. Use of High Doses of Vitamin C in Infections. *Presse Medical,* vol. 55: p. 72. 1947.

28. W. J. McCormick. Vitamin C in the Prophylaxis and Therapy of Infectious Diseases. *Archives of Pediatrics,* vol. 68: pp. 1–9, 1951. Ascorbic Acid as a Chemotherapeutic Agent. Ibid. vol. 69: pp. 151–155. 1952.

29. F. Caels. Contribution to the Study of the Effect of High Doses of Vitamin C in Oto-Rhino-Laryngological Infections.

Acta Oto-Rhino-Laryngologica Belgica (Bruxelles), vol. 7: pp. 395–410. 1953.

30. E. C. Mick. Brucellosis and Its Treatment. *Archives of Pediatrics,* vol. 72: pp. 119–125. 1955.

31. S. Tanabe. Vitamin C Content of Mucous Membranes of Paranasal Sinuses. *Otolaryngology* (Tokyo), vol. 35: pp. 25–30. 1963.

Chapter 15 — Cancer

1. E. L. Kennaway et al. Effect of Aromatic Compounds upon the Ascorbic Acid Content of the Liver in Mice. *Cancer Research,* vol. 4: pp. 367–376. 1944.
   M. Daff et al. Effect of Carcinogenic Compounds on the Ascorbic Acid Content of the Liver in Mice and Rats. *Cancer Research,* vol. 8: pp. 376–380. 1948.
   L. A. Elson et al. Effect of 1:2:5:6 Dibenzanthrene on the Ascorbic Acid Content of the Liver of Rats Maintained on High and Low Protein Diets. *British Journal of Cancer,* vol. 3: pp. 148–156. 1949.
   E. Boyland et al. Stimulation of Ascorbic Acid Synthesis by Carcinogenic and Other Foreign Compounds. *Biochemical Journal,* vol. 81: pp. 163–168. 1961.

2. E. L. Kennaway et al. Carcinogenic Agents and the Metabolism of Ascorbic Acid in the Guinea Pig. *British Journal of Cancer,* vol. 9: pp. 606–610. 1955.

3. W. O. Russell et al. Studies on Methylcholanthrene Induction of Tumors in Scorbutic Guinea Pigs. *Cancer Research,* vol. 12: pp. 216–218. 1952.
   T. R. Miller and B. Sokoloff. A Vitamin C-Free Diet in Radiation Therapy of Malignant Disease. *Journal of Roentgenology,* vol. 73: pp. 472–480. 1955.

4. W. G. Deucher. Vitamin C Metabolism in Tumor Patients. *Strahlentherapie,* vol. 67: pp. 143–151. 1940.
   E. Palenque. On the Treatment of Chronic Myeloid Leukemia with Vitamin C. *Semana Medicà Espanola,* vol. 6: pp. 101–105. 1943.

H. Schirmacher and J. Schneider. Limits and Possibilities of Supervitaminization for Inoperable and X-ray Resistant Carcinoma. *Zeitschrift fur Geburtshilfe und Gyanaekologie* (Stuttgart), vol. 144: pp. 172–182. 1955.

E. Piche and K. Weghaupt. Treatment of Advanced Carcinomas of Female Genitalia with Large Doses of Vitamin A and C. *Wiener Medizinische Wochenschrift*, vol. 106: pp. 391–392. 1956.
S. B. Tagi-Zade. Vitamin C Metabolism in Cancer Patients During Radiotherapy. *Meditsinskaia Radiologiia* (Moskva), vol. 6: pp. 10–16. 1961.
T. Szenes. Effect Of Ascorbic Acid During Roentgen Irradiation Of Tumors. *Strahlentherapie*, vol. 71: pp. 463–471. 1942.

5. L. Benade, T. Howard and D. Burk. Synergistic Killing of Ehrlich Ascites Carcinoma Cells by Ascorbate and 3-Amino-1,2,4-Triazole. *Oncology*, vol. 23: pp. 33–43. 1969.
J. U. Schlegel et al. Studies in the Etiology and Prevention of Bladder Carcinoma. *The Journal of Urology*, vol. 101: pp. 317–324. 1969.

6. von Wendt. *Zeitschrift fur die Gesamte Innere Medizin und Ihre Grenzgebiete* (Stuttgart), vol. 4: 267. 1949. vol. 5: p. 255, 1950. vol. 6: pp. 255-256. 1951. *Hippokrates* (Stuttgart), H. 9, 1951.
L. Huber. Hypervitaminization with Vitamin A and Vitamin C: In Cases of Inoperable Cancer of the Uterus. *Zentralblatt fur Gynaekologie*, vol. 75: pp. 1771–1777. 1953.
E. Schneider. Vitamin C and A in Cancer. *Deutsche Medizinische Wochenschrift*, vol. 79: pp. 584–586. 1954. Mechanism of Resistance to Cancer Shown by a Skin Reaction. *Wiener Medizinische Wochenschrift,* vol. 105: pp. 430–432. 1955. Hypervitamin Therapy of Cancer. *Medizinische*, pp. 183–187. 1956.

7. W. J. McCormick. Cancer: The Preconditioning Factor in Pathogenesis. *Archives of Pediatrics*, vol. 71: pp. 313–322. 1954. Cancer: A Collagen Disease, Secondary to a Nutritional Deficiency? Ibid., vol. 76: pp. 166–171. 1959. Cancer: A Preventable Disease, Secondary to a Nutritional Deficiency. *Clinical Physiology*, vol. 5: pp. 198–204. 1963.

8. A. Goth and I. Littmann. Ascorbic Acid Content in Human Cancer Tissue. *Cancer Research*, vol. 8: pp. 349–351. 1948.

9. F. L. Warren. Aerobic Oxidation of Aromatic Hydrocarbons in Presence of Ascorbic Acid. *Biochemical Journal*, vol. 37: pp. 338–341. 1943.

10. D. J. Stephen and E. E. Hawley. Portion of Reduced Ascorbic Acid in Blood. *Journal of Biological Chemistry*, vol. 115: pp. 653–658. 1936.

11. H. Eufinger and G. Gaehtgens. Effect of Vitamin C on the Pathologic Concentrations of White Blood Cells. *Klinische Wochenschrift*, vol. 15: pp. 150–151. 1936.
H. Schnetz. Vitamin C and Leucocyte Numbers. *Klinische Wochenschrift*, vol. 17: pp. 267–269. 1938.

12. P. Plum and S. Thomsen. Remission in the Course of Aleukemic Leukemia. *Ugeskrift for Laeger* (Kobenhavn), vol. 98: pp. 1062–1067. 1936.
S. Heinild and Schiedt. Remissions During Course of Leukemia Treated with Ascorbic Acid. *Ugeskrift for Laeger* (Kobenhavn), vol. 98: pp. 1135–1136. 1936.
W. Thiele. Effect of Vitamin C on the White Blood Cells and Chronic Myeloid Leukemia. *Klinische Wochenschrift*, vol. 17: pp. 150–151. 1938.
C. L. C. van Nieuwenhuizen. Effect of Vitamin C on the Blood Picture of Patient with Leukemia. *Nederlands Tijdschrift voor Geneeskunde* (Amsterdam), vol. 7: pp. 896–902. 1943.

13. A. Vogt. Vitamin C Treatment of Chronic Leukemias. *Deutsche Medizinische Wochenschrift*, vol. 66: pp. 369–372. 1940.
E. D. Kyhos et al. Large Doses of Ascorbic Acid in Treatment of Vitamin C Deficiencies. *Archives of Internal Medicine*, vol. 75: pp. 407–412. 1945.
A. L. Waldo and R. E. Zipf. Ascorbic Acid Level in Leukemia Patients. *Cancer*, vol. 8: pp. 187–190. 1955.

14. E. Greer. Alcoholic Cirrhosis; Complicated by Polycythemia Vera and then Myelogenous Leukemia and Tolerance of

Large Doses of Vitamin C. *Medical Times* (Manhasset), vol. 82: pp. 865–868. 1954.

Chapter 16 — The Heart, Vascular System, and Strokes

1. J. F. Rinehart and S. R. Mettier. The Heart Valves and Muscle in Experimental Scurvy with Superimposed Infection. *American Journal of Pathology*, vol. 10: pp. 61–79. 1934.

2. M. L. Menten and C. G. King. The Influence of Vitamin C Level upon Resistance to Diptheria Toxin. *Journal of Nutrition*, vol. 10: pp. 141–153. 1935.

3. S. Taylor. Scurvy and Carditis. *Lancet*, vol. 1: pp. 973–979. 1937.

4. J. C. Paterson. Some Factors in the Causation of Intimal Hemorrhages and in the Precipitation of Coronary Thrombi. *Canadian Medical Association Journal*, vol. 44: pp. 114–120. 1941.

5. R. W. Trimmer and C. J. Lundy. A Nutrition Survey in Heart Disease. *American Practitioner*, vol. 2: pp. 448–450. 1948.

6. G. C. Willis. An Experimental Study of the Intimal Ground Substance in Atherosclerosis. *Canadian Medical Association Journal*, vol. 69: pp. 17–22. 1953.

7. G. C. Willis et al. Serial Arteriography in Atherosclerosis. *Canadian Medical Association Journal*, vol. 71: pp. 562–568. 1954.

8. G. C. Willis and S. Fishman. Ascorbic Acid Content of Human Arterial Tissue. *Canadian Medical Association Journal*, vol. 72: pp. 500–503. 1955.

9. W. J. McCormick. Coronary Thrombosis: A New Concept of Mechanism and Etiology. *Clinical Medicine*, pp. 839–845. July 1957.

10. J. Vogel. *The Pathological Anatomy of the Human Body.* Philadelphia: Lea and Blanchard. 1847.

11. N. Anitschkow and S. Chalatow. Ueber Experimentelle Cholesterinsteatese und ihre Bedeutung fur die Entstehung Einigger Pathologischer Prozesse. *Zentralblatt Allgemeine Pathologie,* vol. 24: p. 1. 1913.

12. R. R. Becker et al. Ascorbic Acid Deficiency and Cholesterol Synthesis. *Journal American Chemical Society,* vol. 75: p. 2020. 1953.

13. E. Ginter et al. The Effect of Chronic Hypovitaminosis C on the Metabolism of Cholesterol and Atherogenesis in Guinea Pigs. *Journal of Atherosclerosis Research,* vol. 10: pp. 341–352. 1969.

14. F. M. Dent et al. *American Journal of Physiology,* vol. 163: p. 700. 1950.
    F. M. Dent and W. M. Booker. *Federation Proceedings,* vol. 10: p. 191. 1951.
    W. M. Booker, et al. Cholesterol-Ascorbic Acid Relationship. *American Journal of Physiology,* vol. 189: pp. 335–337. 1957.

15. C. F. Shaffer. Ascorbic Acid and Atherosclerosis. *American Journal of Clinical Nutrition,* vol. 23: pp. 27–30. 1970.

16. V. N. Kolmakov. Effect of Vitamin C on Hypercholesterolemia in Fasting Rabbits. *Voprosy Meditsinskoi Khimii* (Moskva), vol. 3: pp. 414–419. 1957.
    A. L. Myasnikov. Influence of Some Factors on Development of Experimental Cholesterol Atherosclerosis. *Circulation,* vol. 17: pp. 99–113. 1958.
    R. N. Chakravarti et al. Studies in Experimental Atherosclerosis. *Indian Journal of Medical Research,* vol. 45: pp. 315–318. 1957.
    K. K. Datey et al. Ascorbic Acid and Experimental Atherosclerosis. *Journal of the Association of Physicians of India* (Bombay), vol. 16: pp. 567–570. 1968.
    B. Sokoloff et al. Aging, Atherosclerosis and Ascorbic Acid Metabolism. *Journal American Geriatric Society,* vol. 14: pp. 1239–1260. 1966.

17. S. Banerjee and A. Baudyopadhyay. Plasma Lipids in Scurvy: Effect of Ascorbic Acid Supplement and Insulin Treatment. *Proceedings Society Experimental Biology and Medicine,* vol. 112: pp. 372–374. 1963.
    E. Ginter et al. Influence of Chronic Vitamin C Deficiency on Composition of Blood Serum. *Journal of Nutrition,* vol. 99: pp. 261–269. 1969.

18. C. Sitaramayya and T. Ali. Studies on Experimental Hypercholesterolemia and Atherosclerosis. *Indian Journal of Physiology and Pharmacology* (Lucknow), vol. 6: pp. 192–204. 1962.

19. K. R. Sebrov. Prophylaxis and Treatment of Arteriosclerosis with Ascorbic Acid. *Terapevticheskii Arkhiv* (Moskva), vol. 28: pp. 58–65. 1956.
    V. T. Uverskaia. Influence of Ascorbic Acid on Cholesterolemia and Acid-Base Balance in Patients with Hypertensive Disease and Atherosclerosis. *Trudy Leningradskogo Sanitarnogigienicheskogo Meditsinskego Instituta,* vol. 40: pp. 150–158. 1958.
    E. P. Federova. Long Term Ascorbic Acid Therapy for Patients with Coronary Atherosclerosis. *Sovetskaia Meditsina* (Moskva), vol. 25: pp. 56–60. 1960.
    L. A. Tiapina. The Effect of Ascorbic Acid on Blood Lipids in Essential Hypertension and Atherosclerosis. *Cor et Vasa* (Praha), vol. 3: pp. 98–106. 1961.
    J. T. Anderson and A. Keys. Safflower Oil, Hydrogenated Safflower Oil and Ascorbic Acid Effects on Serum Cholesterol in Man. *Federation Proceedings* (Bethesda), vol. 16: p. 380. 1957.
    A. Cortinovis et al. Ascorbic Acid and Atherosclerosis. *Giornale di Gerontologia* (Firenze), vol. 8: pp. 28–31. 1960.
    B. Sokoloff et al. Effect of Ascorbic Acid on Certain Blood Fat Metabolism Factors in Animals and Man. *Journal of Nutrition,* vol. 91: pp. 107–118. 1967.

20. G. C. Willis. The Reversibility of Atherosclerosis. *Canadian Medical Association Journal,* vol. 77: pp. 106–109. 1957.
    R. O. Mumma. Ascorbic Acid as a Sulfating Agent. *Biochimica et Biophysica Acta,* vol. 165: pp. 571–573. 1968.

R. O. Mumma et al. L-Ascorbic Acid 3-Sulfate, Preparation and Characterization. *Carbohydrate Research,* vol. 19: pp. 127–132. 1971.

R. O. Mumma and A. J. Verlangieri. In Vivo Sulfation of Cholesterol by Ascorbic Acid 3-Sulfate as a Possible Explanation for the Hypocholestemic Effects of Ascorbic Acid. *Federation Proceedings,* vol. 30, No. 2, March-April 1971.

C. R. Spittle. Atherosclerosis and Vitamin C. *Lancet,* vol. 2· pp. 1280–1281. 1971.

E. M. Baker, III. Ascorbate Sulfate: A Urinary Metabolite of Ascorbic Acid in Man. *Science,* vol. 173: pp. 826–827. 1971.

21. S. Lindsay and I. L. Chaikoff. Naturally Occurring Arteriosclerosis in Non-Human Primates. *Journal Atherosclerosis Research,* vol. 61: pp. 36–61. 1966.

22. C. Sitaramayya and T. Ali. Studies on Experimental Hypercholesterolemia and Atherosclerosis. *Indian Journal of Physiology and Pharmacology,* vol. 6: pp. 192–204. 1962.

23. R. Tislowitz. *Comptes Rendus des Séances dela Société Biologie et de Ses Filiales* (Paris), vol. 121: pp. 914–916. 1936.

M. A. Abbasy. The Diuretic Action of Vitamin C. *Biochemical Journal,* vol. 31: pp. 339–342. 1937.

24. W. Evans. Vitamin C in Heart Failure. *Lancet,* vol. 1: pp. 308–309. 1938.

25. C. F. Shaffer. The Diuretic Effect of Ascorbic Acid. *Journal American Medical Association,* vol. 124: pp. 700–701. 1944. Ascorbic Acid as a Diuretic. *Lancet,* vol. 2: p. 186. 1944.

C. F. Shaffer et al. The Use of Oral Mercuhydrin Combined with Ascorbic Acid in Cardiac Decompensation. *American Journal Medical Sciences,* vol. 219: pp. 674–678. 1950.

M. R. Kenawy et al. Studies on the Diuretic Action of Vitamin C in Normal Animals and Human Beings and Its Clinical Value in Pathological Retention of Water. *Internationale Zeitschrift fur Vitaminforschung* (Bern), vol. 24: pp. 40–61. 1952.

26. I. M. Scheinker. Changes in Cerebral Veins in Hypertensive

Brain Disease and Their Relation to Cerebral Hemorrhage. *Archives of Neurology and Psychiatry,* vol. 54: pp. 395–408. 1945.

27. E. T. Gale and M. W. Thewlis. Vitamin C and P in Cardiovascular and Cerebrovascular Disease. *Geriatrics,* vol. 8: pp. 80–87. 1953.

28. I. Stone. On the Genetic Etiology of Scurvy. *Acta Geneticae Medicae et Gemellologiae,* vol. 15: pp. 345–350. 1966.

Chapter 17 — Arthritis and Rheumatism

1. Arthritis. Public Health Service Publication No. 1444-A, U. S. Department of Health, Education and Welfare, Washington, D. C. April 1966.

2. J. M. Rivers. Ascorbic Acid in Metabolism of Connective Tissue. *New York State Journal of Medicine,* vol. 65: pp. 1235-1238. 1965.

3. W. V. Robertson. The Biochemical Role of Ascorbic Acid in Connective Tissue. *Annals New York Academy of Sciences,* vol. 92: pp. 159–167. 1961.

4. S. Udenfriend. Formation of Hydroxyproline in Collagen. *Science,* vol. 152: pp. 1335–1340. 1966.

5. N. Stone and A. Meister. Function of Ascorbic Acid in the Conversion of the Proline to Collagen Hydroxyproline. *Nature,* vol. 194: p. 555. 1962.

6. J. F. Rinehart. Further Observations on Pathologic Similarities between Experimental Scurvy Combined with Infection and Rheumatic Fever. *Journal of Experimental Medicine,* vol. 59: pp. 97–114 (with 11 Plates). 1934.
   J. F. Rinehart. Studies Relating Vitamin C Deficiency to Rheumatic Fever and Rheumatoid Arthritis: Experimental, Clinical and General Considerations. I. Rheumatic Fever. *Annals Internal Medicine,* vol. 9: pp. 586–599. 1935. II. Rheumatoid (Atrophic) Arthritis, Ibid. vol. 9: pp. 671–689. 1935.

J. F. Rinehart. An Outline of Studies Relating Vitamin C Deficiency in Rheumatic Fever. *Journal of Laboratory and Clinical Medicine*, vol. 21: pp. 597–608. 1936.

J. F. Rinehart et al. Reduced Ascorbic Acid Content of Blood Plasma in Rheumatoid Arthritis. *Proceedings Society Experimental Biology and Medicine*, vol. 35: pp. 347-352. 1936.

J. F. Rinehart. Vitamin C and Rheumatic Fever. *International Clinics*, vol. 2: pp. 22–35. 1937.

J. F. Rinehart, et al. Metabolism of Vitamin C in Rheumatoid Arthritis. *Archives of Internal Medicine*, vol. 61: pp. 537–561. 1938.

7. M. A. Abbasy et al. Vitamin C and Juvenile Rheumatism. *Lancet*, vol. 2: pp. 1413–1417. 1936.

L. J. Harris et al. Vitamin C and Infection. *Lancet*, vol. 2: pp. 177–180. 1937.

M. A. Abbasy et al. Excretion of Vitamin C in Pulmonary Tuberculosis and in Rheumatoid Arthritis. *Lancet*, vol. 2: pp. 181–183. 1937.

L. J. Harris et al. Influence of Infection on the Vitamin C Content of the Tissues of Animals. *Lancet*, vol. 2: pp. 183–186. 1937.

G. Mouriquand et al. Osteoses and Penosteoses from Chronic Dietary Deficiencies. *Presse Médicale*, No. 81: pp. 1419–1420. October 9, 1937.

A. D. Kaiser. Rheumatic Infection: Is Vitamin C Deficiency a Factor? *New York State Journal of Medicine*, vol. 38: pp. 868–873. 1938.

A. D. Kaiser and B. Slavin. The Incidence of Hemolytic Streptococci in the Tonsils of Children as Related to the Vitamin C Content of Tonsils and Blood. *Journal of Pediatrics*, vol. 13: pp. 322–333. 1938.

A. K. Sherwood. Vitamin C and Arthritis. *Northwest Medicine*, vol. 37: pp. 288–289. 1938.

T. Mouriquand. Chronic Rheumatism and Avitaminosis. *Annales de Médecine*, vol. 46: pp. 249–266. 1939–40.

8. C. B. Perry. Rheumatic Heart Disease and Vitamin C. *Lancet*, vol. 2: pp. 426–427. 1935.

M. P. Schultz. Cardiovascular and Arthritic Lesions in

Guinea Pigs with Chronic Scurvy and Hemolytic Streptococcic Infections. *Archives of Pathology,* vol. 21: pp. 472–495. 1936.

J. Sendroy, Jr., and M. P. Schultz. Studies of Ascorbic Acid and Rheumatic Fever. *Journal of Clinical Investigation,* vol. 15: pp. 369–383. 1936.

9. M. P. Schultz. Studies on Ascorbic Acid and Rheumatic Fever. II. Test of Prophylactic and Therapeutic Action of Ascorbic Acid. *Journal of Clinical Investigation,* vol. 15: pp. 385–391. 1936.

10. F. H. Mosse. A Case of Rheumatic Fever Treated with Vitamin C. *Chinese Medical Journal,* vol. 53: pp. 72–77. 1938.

11. M. G. Hall et al. The Vitamin C Requirement in Rheumatoid Arthritis. *Annals Internal Medicine,* vol. 13: pp. 415–423. 1939.

12. R. H. Jacques. Relation Between Reduced Ascorbic Acid Levels of the Blood Plasma and Rheumatoid Arthritis. *Journal of Bone and Joint Surgery,* vol. 22: pp. 324–326. 1940.

13. I. M. Vilyanski. Ascorbic Acid Therapy and Acute Articular Rheumatism. *Klinicheskaia Meditsina* (Moskva), vol. 19: p. 121. 1941.

14. R. H. Freyberg. Treatment of Arthritis with Vitamin and Endocrine Preparations. Emphasis of Their Limited Value. *Journal American Medical Association,* vol. 119: pp. 1165–1167. 1942.

15. E. F. Trant and F. L. Matousek. The Relation of Ascorbic Acid to Chronic Arthritis. *Illinois Medical Journal,* vol. 95: pp. 38–39. 1949.

16. J. F. Rinehart. Rheumatic Fever and Nutrition. *Annals Rheumatic Diseases* (London), vol. 3: pp. 154–167. 1943.

17. B. F. Massell. Antirheumatic Activity of Ascorbic Acid in Large Doses. *New England Journal of Medicine,* vol. 242: pp. 614–615. 1950.

18. H. Baufeld. Ascorbic Acid in the Treatment of Polyarthritis. *Deutsche Gesundheitswesen* (Berlin), vol. 7: p. 1077. 1952.

19. E. Greer. A Current Case of Rheumatic Fever. *Medical Times*, vol. 81: pp. 483–484. 1953.

20. W. J. McCormick. The Rheumatic Diseases: Is There a Common Etiologic Factor? *Archives of Pediatrics*, vol. 72: pp. 107–112. 1955.

21. E. K. Afanasieva. The Role of Ascorbic Acid in the Prophylaxis and Therapy of Rheumatic Fever. *Trudy Leningradskogo Sanitarnogigienicheskogo Meditsinskogo Instituta*, vol. 48: pp. 34–43. 1959.

Chapter 18 — Aging

1. J. Bjorksten. Dr. Shannon Is Unhappy. *The Chemist*, pp. 377–379. October 1965.
   J. Bjorksten. Aging, Primary Mechanism. *Gerontologia*, vol. 8: pp. 179–192. 1963.

2. I. Stone. The Genetic Disease Hypoascorbemia. A Fresh Approach to an Ancient Disease and Some of Its Medical Implications. *Acta Geneticae Medicae et Gemellologiae*, vol. 16: pp. 52–62. 1967.

3. F. Verzár. The Aging of Collagen. *Scientific American*, p. 104. April 1963.
   J. Bjorksten. Aging: Present Status of Our Chemical Knowledge. *Journal American Geriatric Society*, vol. 10: pp. 125–139. 1962.
   F. M. Sinex. Biochemistry of Aging. *Science*, vol. 134: pp 1402–1405. 1961.
   D. Harman. Aging: A Theory Based on Free Radical and Radiation Chemistry. *Journal of Gerontology*, vol. 11: pp. 298–300. 1952.
   I. G. Fels. Molecular Aging and Senescence. *Gerontologia*, vol. 12: pp. 109–121. 1966.
   W. Reichel. The Biology of Aging. *Journal of the American Geriatrics Society*, vol. 14: pp. 431–446. 1960.

4. F. M. Sinex. Aging and the Lability of Irreplaceable Mole-

cules. *Journal of Gerontology*, vol. 12: pp. 191–197. 1957.

A. Aslan and A. Vrabiesco. A Study of the Evolution in Regard to Age of Certain Physical Constants of Collagen. *Gerontologia*, vol. 11: pp. 34–44. 1965.

F. Verzár and H. Spichtin. The Role of the Pituitary in Aging of Collagen. *Gerontologia*, vol. 12: pp. 48–56. 1966.

C. D. Nordschow. Aspects of Aging in Human Collagen: An Exploratory Thermoelastic Study. *Experimental and Molecular Pathology*, vol. 5: pp. 350–373. 1966.

R. Goodman. Speculations on Vascular Changes With Age. *Journal of the American Geriatrics Society*, vol. 18: pp. 765–779. 1970.

5. A. L. Tappel. Will Antioxidant Nutrients Slow Aging Processes? *Geriatrics*, vol. 23: pp. 97–105. 1968.

6. A. Comfort. Gerontology: Antioxidants Slow Aging. *Chemical and Engineering News*, p. 13. September 1, 1969.

7. B. Sokoloff et al. Aging, Atherosclerosis and Ascorbic Acid Metabolism. *Journal of the American Geriatrics Society*. vol. 14: pp. 1239–1260. 1966.

8. M. Yavorsky et al. The Vitamin C Content of Human Tissues. *Journal of Biological Chemistry*, vol. 106: pp. 525–529. 1934.

H. A. Rafsky and B. Newman. Vitamin C Studies in the Aged. *American Journal of Medical Sciences*. vol. 201: pp. 749–756. 1941.

M. W. Thewlis and E. T. Gale. Nutrition in the Aged. *Journal of the American Institute of Homeopathy*, vol. 40: pp. 266–268. 1947.

H. D. Chope. Relation of Nutrition to Health in Aging Persons. *California Medicine*, vol. 81: pp. 335–338. 1954.

H. D. Chope and L. Breslow. Nutritional Status of the Aging. *American Journal of Public Health*, vol. 46: pp. 61–67. 1956.

A. F. Morgan. Nutritional Status of Aging. *Journal of Nutrition*, vol. 55: pp. 431–448. 1955.

9. K. W. Denson and E. F. Bowers. The Determination of Ascorbic Acid in White Blood Cells. *Clinical Science*, vol. 21: pp. 157–162. 1961.

E. F. Bowers and M. M. Kubik. Vitamin C Levels in Old

People and the Response to Ascorbic Acid. *British Journal of Clinical Practice,* vol. 19: pp. 141–147. 1965.

B. I. Smolianski. Vitamin C. Requirements in Early and Advanced Old Age. *Voprosy Pitanii* (Moskva), vol. 24: pp. 23–26. 1965.

J. Andrews and M. Brook. Leucocyte-Vitamin C Content and Clinical Signs in the Elderly. *Lancet,* vol. 1: pp. 1350–1351. 1966.

J. Andrews et al. Influence of Abode and Season on the Vitamin C Status of the Elderly. *Gerontologia Clinica* (Basel), vol. 8: pp. 257–266. 1966.

D. J. O'Sullivan, et al. Ascorbic Acid Deficiency in the Elderly. *Irish Journal of Medical Science,* vol. 1: pp. 151–156. 1968.

M. L. Mitra. Vitamin C Deficiency in the Elderly and Its Manifestations. *Journal American Geriatrics Society,* vol. 18: pp. 67–71. 1970.

10. G. E. Slotkin and R. S. Fletcher. Ascorbic Acid in Pulmonary Complications Following Prostatic Surgery: A Preliminary Report. *Journal of Urology,* vol. 52: pp. 566–569. 1944.

11. B. L. Smolyanskii. Effect of Ascorbic Acid on Functional State of Adrenal Cortex in Elderly Persons. *Terapevticheskii Arkhiv,* vol. 35: pp. 71–77. 1963.

B. K. Patnaik. Change in the Bound Ascorbic Acid Content of Muscle and Liver of Rats in Relation to Age. *Nature,* vol. 218: p. 393. 1968.

Chapter 19 — Allergies, Asthma, and Hay Fever

1. S. Raffel and R. R. Madison. The Influence of Ascorbic Acid on Anaphylaxis in Guinea Pigs. *Journal of Infectious Diseases,* vol. 63: pp. 71–76. 1938.

M. Walzer. A Critical Review of the Recent Literature on Vitamin C in Relation to Hypersensitiveness. *Journal of Allergy,* vol. 10: pp. 72–94. 1938.

2. G. Pacheco and M. Para. Vitamine C et Anaphylaxie.

Comptes Rendus des Séances de la Société de Biologie et de Ses Filiales, vol. 129: pp. 419–421. 1938.

K. Yoshikawa. On the Antiallergic Effect of Vitamin C. *Nagasaki Igakkai Zassi*, vol. 17: pp. 165–168. 1938.

3. S. Yokoyama. On the Influence of Vitamine C on Anaphylactic Shock. *Kitasato Archives of Experimental Medicine*, vol. 17: pp. 17–37. 1940.

H. M. Guirgis. Anti-anaphylactic Effect of Vitamin C in the Guinea Pig. *Journal of Pharmacy and Pharmacology*, vol. 17: p. 387. 1965.

W. Dawson and G. B. West. The Influence of Ascorbic Acid on Histamine Metabolism in Guinea Pigs. *British Journal of Pharmacology*, vol. 24: pp. 725–734. 1965.

4. B. Csaba and S. Toth. The Effect of Ascorbic Acid on Anaphylactic Shock in Dogs. *Journal of Pharmacy and Pharmacology*, vol. 18: p. 325. 1966.

H. Herxheimer. Protection against Anaphylactic Shock by Various Substances. *British Journal of Pharmacology*, vol. 10: pp. 160–163. 1955.

5. H. N. Holmes and W. Alexander. Hay Fever and Vitamin C. *Science*, vol. 96: pp. 497–499. 1942.

H. N. Holmes. Food Allergies and Vitamin C. *Annals of Allergy*, vol. 1: p. 235. 1943.

R. Korbsch. Cevitamic Acid Therapy of Allergic Inflammatory Conditions. *Medizinische Klinik*, vol. 34: p. 1500. 1938.

6. L. Pelner. The Importance of Vitamin C in Bodily Defenses. *Annals of Allergy*, vol. 2: pp. 231–232. 1944.

L. Pelner. Sensitivity to Sulfonamide Compounds Avoided by Combined Use with Ascorbic Acid. *New York State Journal of Medicine*, vol. 43: p. 1874. 1943.

L. Pelner. The Effect of Ascorbic Acid in the Sensitivity to Salicylates in a Case of Rheumatic Fever. *Journal of Laboratory and Clinical Medicine*, vol. 28: pp. 28-30. 1942.

7. S. Hebald. Clinical Evaluation of Ascorbic Acid in the Treatment of Hay Fever. *Journal of Allergy*, vol. 15: pp. 236–238. 1944.

D. L. Engelsher. Questionable Value of Vitamin C for Hay

Fever. *Journal American Medical Association,* vol. 126: p. 318. 1944.

8. S. Ruskin. High Dosage Vitamin C in Allergy. *American Journal of Digestive Diseases,* vol. 12: pp. 281–313. 1945.
   S. Friedlander and S. M. Feinberg. Vitamin C in Hay Fever: Therapy and Blood Levels. *Journal of Allergy,* vol. 16: pp. 140–145. 1945.

9. S. Ruskin. Sodium Ascorbate in the Treatment of Allergic Disburbances. *The American Journal of Digestive Diseases,* vol. 14: pp. 302–306. 1947.
   S. Ruskin. The Epinephrine Potenticity Effect of Sodium Ascorbate in Allergy. *Eye, Ear, Nose and Throat Monthly,* vol. 27: pp. 63–69. 1948.
   E. A. Brown and S. Ruskin. The Use of Cevitamic Acid in the Symptomatic and Coseasonal Treatment of Pollinosis. *Annals of Allergy,* vol. 7: pp. 65–70. 1949.

10. G. A. Goldsmith et al. Vitamin C (Ascorbic Acid) Nutrition in Bronchial Asthma. *Archives of Internal Medicine,* vol. 67: pp. 597–608. 1941.
    N. B. Silbert. Vitamin C. Critical Review. *Medical Times,* vol. 79: pp. 370–376. 1951.

11. W. Dawson and G. B. West. The Nature of the Antagonism of Bronchospasm in the Guinea Pig by Ascorbic Acid. *Journal of Pharmacy and Pharmacology,* vol. 17: pp. 595-596, 1965. W. Dawson et al. Actions of Sodium Ascorbate on Smooth Muscle. *British Journal Pharmacology and Chemotherapeutics,* vol. 31: pp. 269–275. 1967.

Chapter 20 — Eye Conditions

1. H. Heath. Distribution and Possible Functions of Ascorbic Acid in the Eye. *Experimental Eye Research,* vol. 1: pp. 362–367. 1962.

2. E. Linnér. Intraocular Pressure Regulation and Ascorbic Acid. *Acta Societatis Medicorum Upsaliensis* (Stockholm), vol. 69: pp. 225–232. 1964.
   E. Linnér. The Pressure Lowering Effect of Ascorbic Acid

in Ocular Hypertension. *Acta Ophthalmologica*, vol. 47: pp. 685–689. 1969.

3. M. Virno et al. Sodium Ascorbate as an Osmotic Agent to Reduce Intracranial and Intraocular Pressures. *Policlinico Sezione Pratica* (Rome), vol. 72: pp. 1746–1752. 1965.
M. Virno et al. Sodium Ascorbate as an Osmotic Agent in Glaucoma. *Bollettino d'Oculistica* (Bologna), vol. 44: pp. 542–550. 1965.
M. Virno et al. Intravenous Glycerol-Vitamin C (Sodium Salt) as Osmotic Agents to Reduce Intraocular Pressure. *American Journal of Ophthalmology*, vol. 62: pp. 824–833. 1966.
M. Virno et al. Oral Treatment of Glaucoma with Vitamin C. *The Eye, Ear, Nose and Throat Monthly*, vol. 46: pp. 1502–1508. 1967.
M. Virno et al. Hypotensive Intraocular Effects of High Oral Doses of Ascorbic Acid in Glaucoma Therapy. *Bollettino d'Oculistica* (Bologna), vol. 46: pp. 259–274. 1967.

4. G. B. Bietti. The Value of Osmotic Hypotonizing Means for the Treatment of Ocular Hypertension. *Transactions Ophthalmological Societies United Kingdom*, vol. 86: pp. 247–254. 1966.
G. B. Bietti. Further Contributions on the Value of Osmotic Substances as Means to Reduce Intra-Ocular Pressure. *Transactions Ophthalmological Society of Australia*, vol. 26: pp. 61–71. 1967.
A. Missiroli et al. Therapeutic Possibilities of Oral Glycerol-Ascorbic Acid in Treatment of Glaucoma. *Bollettino d'Oculistica* (Bologna), vol. 46: pp. 877–890. 1967.
R. Neuschuler et al. Retinal Arterial Pressure in Normal Subjects with Oral Glycerol and Intravenous Sodium Ascorbate. *Bollettino d'Oculistica*, vol. 46: pp. 865–876. 1967.
A. Missiroli et al. Ocular Tension and Ascorbic Acid Content of Aqueous Humor. *Bollettino d'Oculistica*, vol. 47: pp. 32–40. 1968.
J. Pecori Giraldi et al. Ascorbic Acid Content of Aqueous Humor and Blood Serum after Oral Administration of Vitamin C to Rabbits. *Bollettino d'Oculistica*, vol. 47: pp. 227–234. 1968.
G. B. Bietti. Vitamin C as an Intraocular Pressure Lowering

Agent. *Bericht*; *Deutsche Ophthalmologische Gesellschaft* (München), vol. 68: pp. 190-206. 1968.

5. C. Hilsdorf. On the Decrease in Intraocular Pressure with Intravenous Sodium Ascorbate. *Monatsblatter fur Augenheilkunde*, vol. 150: pp. 352–358. 1967.
R. Esila et al. Effect of Ascorbic Acid on Intraocular Pressure and Aqueous Humor of Rabbit Eye. *Acta Ophthalmologica* (Kobenhavn), vol. 44: pp. 631–636. 1966.

6. Summary of Progress in Eye Disorders. Revised 1966. Public Health Service Publication No. 1155, U. S. Department of Health, Education and Welfare, Washington, D. C., p. 5.

7. Eye Lenses Are Made Up of Protein Helixes. *Chemical and Engineering News*, p. 44. April 5, 1965.

8. Z. Dische and H. Zil. Studies on the Oxidation of Cysteine to Cystine in Lens Proteins during Cataract Formation. *American Journal of Ophthalmology*, vol. 38: pp. 104–113. 1951.

9. H. V. Nema and S. P. Srivastava. Ascorbic Acid in Aqueous and Serum in Normal and Mature Cataractous Indian Patients. *Journal All-India Ophthalmological Society*, vol. 11: pp. 58–61. 1963.
D. P. Sinha and K. P. Sinha. Observations on Glutathione and Ascorbic Acid Content in Human and Cataractous Lens. *Journal Indian Medical Association*, vol. 46: pp. 646–649. 1966.
R. N. Consul and P. N. Nagpal. Quantitative Study of the Variations in the Levels of Glutathione and Ascorbic Acid in Human Lenses with Senile Cataract. *The Eye, Ear, Nose and Throat Monthly*, vol. 47: pp. 336–339. 1968.

10. T. K. Lyle and D. W. McLean. Vitamin C (Ascorbic Acid)—Its Therapeutic Value in Inflammatory Conditions of the Cornea. *British Journal of Ophthalmology*, vol. 25: pp. 286–295. 1941.
T. C. Summers. Penicillin and Vitamin C in the Treatment of Hypopyon Ulcer. *British Journal of Ophthalmology*, vol. 30: pp. 128–134. 1946.
T. A. S. Boyd and F. W. Campbell. Influence of Ascorbic

Acid on the Healing of Corneal Ulcers in Man. *British Medical Journal,* vol. 2: pp. 1145–1148. 1950.

F. W. Campbell and I. D. Ferguson. The Role of Ascorbic Acid in Corneal Vascularization. *British Journal of Ophthalmology,* vol. 34: pp. 329-334. 1950.

F. W. Campbell et al. Ascorbic Acid and Healing of Heat Injuries in the Guinea Pig Cornea. *British Journal of Nutrition,* vol. 4: pp. 32–42. 1950.

T. A. S. Boyd. Influence of Local Ascorbic Acid Concentrations on the Collagenous Tissue Healing in the Cornea. *British Journal of Ophthalmology,* vol. 39: pp. 204–214. 1955.

11. V. Muhlmann et al. Vitamin C Therapy of Incipient Senile Cataract. *Archives de Oftalmologia de Buenos Aires,* vol. 14: pp. 552–575. 1939.

    S. M. Bouton, Jr. Vitamin C and the Aging Eye. *Archives of Internal Medicine,* vol. 63: pp. 930–945. 1939.

    D. T. Atkinson. Malnutrition as an Etiological Factor in Senile Cataract. *The Eye, Ear, Nose and Throat Monthly,* vol. 31: pp. 79–83. 1952.

12. G. Erlanger. Iontophoresis, a Scientific and Practical Tool in Ophthalmology. *Ophthalmologica,* vol. 128: pp. 232–246. 1954.

13. J. C. Weber and F. M. Wilson. Biochemical Studies of Subretinal Fluid. *Archives of Ophthalmology,* vol. 71: pp. 556–557. 1964.

Chapter 21 — Ulcers

1. D. T. Smith and M. McConkey. Peptic Ulcers (Gastric, Pyloric and Duodenal): Occurrence in Guinea Pigs on a Diet Deficient in Vitamin C. *Archives of Internal Medicine,* vol. 51: pp. 413–426. 1933.

   H. Hanke. The Role of Vitamin C Deficiency in Gastric Ulcers. *Deutsche Zeitschrift fur Chirurgie,* vol. 249: pp. 213–223. 1937.

2. H. E. Archer and George Graham. The Subscurvy State in Relation to Gastric and Duodenal Ulcer. *Lancet,* vol. 2: pp. 364–367. 1936.

T. H. Ingalls and H. A. Warren. Asymptomatic Scurvy. Its Relation to Wound Healing and Its Incidence in Patients with Peptic Ulcer. *New England Journal of Medicine,* vol. 217: pp. 443–446. 1937.

B. Portnoy and J. F. Wilkinson. Vitamin C Deficiency in Peptic Ulceration and Haematemosis. *British Medical Journal,* vol. 1: pp. 554–560. 1938.

H. A. Warren et al. Ascorbic Acid Requirements in Patients with Peptic Ulcer. *New England Journal of Medicine,* vol. 220: pp. 1061–1063. 1939.

H. Field, Jr. et al. Vitamins in Peptic Ulcer. *Annals of Internal Medicine,* vol. 14: pp. 588-592. 1940.

J. B. Ludden et al. Studies on Ascorbic Acid Deficiency in Gastric Diseases: Incidence, Diagnosis and Treatment. *American Journal of Digestive Diseases,* vol. 8: pp. 249–252. 1941.

J. H. Roe et al. The Relation of Nutrition to Gastric Function, II. The Effect of Vitamin C Deficiency. *American Journal of Digestive Diseases,* vol. 8: pp. 261–266. 1941.

V. M. Crescenzo and D. Cayer. Plasma Vitamin C Levels in Patients with Peptic Ulcer. *Gastroenterology,* vol. 8: pp. 757–761. 1947.

L. A. Rosenblum. Management of Peptic Ulcer with Unrestricted Diet and a New Combination of Therapeutic Agents. *The American Journal of Gastroenterology,* vol. 28: pp. 507–517. 1957.

E. C. Nash. A Comparative Study of an Antacid with and without Vitamin C in the Treatment of Peptic Ulcer. *American Practitioner and Digest of Treatments,* vol. 3: pp. 117–120. 1952.

C. Debray et al. Treatment of Gastro-Duodenal Ulcers with Large Doses of Ascorbic Acid. *Semaine Thérapeutique* (Paris), vol. 44: pp. 393–398. 1968.

R. L. Russell et al. Ascorbic Acid Levels in Leucocytes of Patients with Gastrointestinal Hemorrhage. *Lancet,* vol. 2: pp. 603–606. 1968.

3. J. Nasio. Effect of Ascorbic Acid upon Cinchophen Experimental Peptic Ulcer. *The Review of Gastroenterology,* vol. 14: pp. 340–344. 1947.

E. Aron. Protective Effect of Ascorbic Acid on Drug Induced Peptic Ulcers. *Thérapie* (Paris), vol. 13: pp. 185–190. 1958.

R. I. Russell and A. Goldberg. Effect of Aspirin on the Gastric Mucosa of Guinea Pigs on a Scorbutogenic Diet. *Lancet*, vol. 2: pp. 606–608. 1968.

4. S. Lazarus. Vitamin C Nutrition in Haematemesis and Malaena. *British Medical Journal*, vol. 2: pp. 1011–1015. 1937.

E. deJ. Zerbini. Vitamin C in Gastric Resection for Peptic Ulcer. *Archives of Surgery*, vol. 54: pp. 117–120. 1947.

J. M. Williamson et al. Leucocyte Ascorbic Acid Levels in Patients with Malabsorption or Previous Gastric Surgery. *British Medical Journal*, vol. 2: pp. 23–25. 1967.

M. M. Cohen. Leucocyte Ascorbic Acid Levels. *British Medical Journal*, vol. 2: p. 243. 1967.

W. P. Small and W. Sircus. Leucocyte Ascorbic Acid Levels. *British Medical Journal*, vol. 2: pp. 375–376 1967.

Malabsorption, Gastric Surgery and Ascorbic Acid *Nutrition Reviews*, vol. 25: pp. 237–239. 1967.

M. M. Cohen and A. M. Duncan. Ascorbic Acid Nutrition in Gastroduodenal Disorders. *British Medical Journal*, vol. 4: pp. 516–518. 1967.

R. Esposito and R. Valentini. Vitamin C and Gastroduodenal Disorders. *British Medical Journal*, vol. 5: p. 118. 1968.

5. Peptic Ulcer. Public Health Service Publication No. 280, Revised 1965, U. S Department of Health, Education and Welfare, Washington, D. C.

The Medical Letter on Drugs and Therapeutics, vol. 11, No. 26, December 26, 1969. Drug and Therapeutic Information Inc., 305 East 45 Street, New York, N.Y. 10017.

Chapter 22 — Kidneys and Bladder

1. J. U. Schlegel et al. The Role of Ascorbic Acid in the Prevention of Bladder Tumor Formation. *Transactions of the American Association of Genito-Urinary Surgeons*, vol. 61: pp. 85–89. 1969.

J. U. Schlegel et al. Studies in the Etiology and Prevention of Bladder Carcinoma. *Journal of Urology,* vol. 101: pp. 317–324. 1969.

2. P. Dite et al. Changes in Plasma Levels of Vitamin C during Hemodialysis in Patients with Chronic Uremia. *La Tunisie Médicale,* vol. 46: pp. 329-335. 1968.

   J. F. Sullivan and A. B. Eisenstein. Ascorbic Acid Depletion in Patients Undergoing Chronic Hemodialysis. *The American Journal of Clinical Nutrition,* vol. 23: pp. 1339–1346. 1970.

   M. F. Mason et al. Effect of p-Aminobenzoic Acid and Vitamin C upon Duration of Survival of Nephrectomized Rats. *Proceedings Society Experimental Biology and Medicine,* vol. 75: pp. 303–304. 1950.

3. S. N. Gershoff. The Formation of Urinary Stones. *Metabolism,* vol. 13: pp. 875–887. 1964.

   K. Lonsdale. Human Stones. *Science,* vol. 159: pp. 1199–1207. 1968.

4. W. J. McCormick. Lithogenesis and Hypovitaminosis. *Medical Record,* vol. 159: pp. 410–413. 1946.

5. M. Frank et al. Prevention of Urolithiasis. *Archives of Environmental Health,* vol. 13: pp. 625–630. 1966.

6. M. P. Lamden and G. A. Chrystowski. Urinary Oxalate Excretion by Man Following Ascorbic Acid Ingestion, *Proceedings Society Experimental Biology and Medicine,* vol. 85: pp. 190–192. 1954.

   K. Takenouchi et al. On the Metabolites of Ascorbic Acid, Especially Oxalic Acid, Eliminated in Urine, Following Administration of Large Amounts of Ascorbic Acid. *Journal of Vitaminology,* vol. 12: pp. 49-58. 1966.

   H. Takaguchi et al. Urinary Oxalic Acid Excretion by Man Following Ingestion of Large Amounts of Ascorbic Acid. *Journal of Vitaminology,* vol. 12: pp. 307-312. 1966.

   M. El-Dakhakhny and M. El-Sayed. The Effect of Some Drugs on Oxalic Excretion in Urine. *Arzneimittel-Forschung* (Aulendorf), vol. 20: pp. 264–267. 1970.

Chapter 23 — Diabetes and Hypoglycemia

1. O. A. Bessey et al. Pathologic Changes in the Organs of Scorbutic Guinea Pigs. *Proceedings Society for Experimental Biology and Medicine*, vol. 31: pp. 455–460. 1934.
A. Sigal and C. G. King. The Relationship of Vitamin C to Glucose Tolerance in the Guinea Pig. *Journal of Biological Chemistry*, vol. 116: pp. 489–492. 1936.
A. Sigal and C. G. King. Influence of Vitamin C Deficiency upon Resistance of Guinea Pigs to Diphtheria Toxin-Glucose Tolerance. *Journal of Pharmacology and Experimental Therapeutics*, vol. 61: p. 1–9. 1937.

2. S. Banerjee. Vitamin C and Carbohydrate Metabolism. *Nature*, vol. 152: p. 329. 1943.
S. Banerjee. Vitamin C and Carbohydrate Metabolism. Part I. Effect of Vitamin C on the Glucose Tolerance Test in Guinea Pigs. *Annals of Biochemistry and Experimental Medicine*, vol. 3: pp. 157–164. 1943.
S. Banerjee. Part II. Effect of Vitamin C on the Glycogen Value of the Liver of Guinea Pigs. *Annals of Biochemistry and Experimental Medicine*, vol. 3: pp. 165–170. 1943.
S. Banerjee. Part IV. Effect of Vitamin C on the Insulin Content of the Pancreas of Guinea Pigs. *Annals of Biochemistry and Experimental Medicine*, vol. 4: pp. 33–36. 1944.
S. Banerjee. Part V. Effect of Vitamin C on the Histology of the Pancreas of Guinea Pigs. *Annals of Biochemistry and Experimental Medicine*, vol. 4: pp. 37-40. 1944.
S. Banerjee and N. C. Ghosh. Relation of Scurvy to Glucose Tolerance Test, Liver Glycogen and Insulin Content of Pancreas of Guinea Pigs. *Journal of Biological Chemistry*, vol. 168: pp. 207–211. 1947.
S. Banerjee et al. Studies on Carbohydrate Metabolism in Scorbutic Guinea Pigs. *Journal of Biological Chemistry*, vol. 230: pp. 261-270. 1958.
S. Banerjee and S. D. Varma. Effect of Scurvy on Active Transport of Glucose by Small Intestine in Vitro. *Proceedings Society Experimental Biology and Medicine*, vol. 116: pp. 216-218. 1964.

3. E. Altenburger. Relationship of Ascorbic Acid on the Storage

and Metabolism of Glycogen in the Liver. *Klinsche Wochenschrift*, vol. 15: pp. 1129–1131. 1936.

C. T. Stewart et al. Factors Determining Effect of Insulin on Metabolism of Glucose in Ascorbic Acid Deficiency and Scurvy in the Monkey. *American Journal of Diseases of Children*, vol. 84: pp. 677–690. 1952.

E. P. Ralli and S. Sherry. Effect of Insulin on Plasma Level and Excretion of Vitamin C. *Proceedings Society Experimental Biology and Medicine*, vol. 43: pp. 669–672. 1940.

S. Sherry and E. P. Ralli. Further Studies of the Effects of Insulin on the Metabolism of Vitamin C. *Journal of Clinical Investigation*, vol. 27: p. 225. 1948.

H. Haid. Vitamin C in Blood in Insulin Shock. *Zeitschrift fur Klinische Medizin*, vol. 139: p. 485. 1941.

E. Wille. Vitamin C and Carbohydrate Metabolism. *Deutsche Medizinische Wochenschrift*, vol. 65: pp. 1117–1120. 1939.

4. H. Bartelheimer. Vitamin C in the Treatment of Diabetes. *Die Medizinische Welt*, vol. 13: 117–120. 1939.

J. M. Rogoff et al. Vitamin C and Insulin Action. *Pennsylvania Medical Journal*, vol. 47: pp. 579–582. 1944.

R. Pfleger and F. Scholl. Diabetes and Vitamin C. *Wiener Archiv fur Innere Medizin*, vol. 31: pp. 219–229. 1937.

5. Editorial. The Tolbutamide Controversy. *Journal American Medical Association*, vol. 213: p. 861. 1970.

6. W. Stepp et al. Vitamin C and Blood Sugar. *Klinische Wochenschrift*, vol. 14: pp. 933–934. 1935.

7. M. G. Goldner and G. Gomori. Production of Diabetes Mellitus in Rats with Alloxan. *Proceedings Society Experimental Biology and Medicine*, vol. 54: p. 287. 1943.

J. W. Patterson. Diabetogenic Effect of Dehydroascorbic Acid. *Endocrinology*, vol. 45: p. 344. 1949.

J. W. Patterson. The Diabetogenic Effect of Dehydroascorbic Acid and Dehydroisoascorbic Acid. *Journal Biological Chemistry*, vol. 183: pp. 81–88. 1950.

J. W. Patterson. Course of Diabetes and Development of Cataracts after Injecting Dehydroascorbic Acid and Related Substances. *American Journal of Physiology*, vol. 165: pp. 61–65. 1951.

S. Levey and B. Suter. Effect of Ascorbic Acid on Diabetogenic Action of Alloxan. *Proceedings Society Experimental Biology and Medicine,* vol. 63: pp. 341–343. 1946.

S. Banerjee. Effect of Scurvy on Glutathione and Dehydroascorbic Acid in Guinea Pig Tissues. *Journal Biological Chemistry,* vol. 195: pp. 271–276. 1952.

8. I. Stone. Studies of a Mammalian Enzyme System for Producing Evolutionary Evidence on Man. *American Journal of Physical Anthropology,* vol. 23: pp. 83–85. 1965.

I. Stone. On the Genetic Etiology of Scurvy. *Acta Geneticae Medicae et Gemollologiae,* vol. 15: pp. 345–349. 1966.

I. Stone. The Genetic Disease, Hypoascorbemia: A Fresh Approach to an Ancient Disease and Some of Its Medical Implications. *Acta Geneticae Medicae et Gemollologiae,* vol. 16: pp. 52–62. 1967.

I. Stone. Hypoascorbemia: The Genetic Disease Causing the Human Requirement for Exogenous Ascorbic Acid. *Perspectives in Biology and Medicine,* vol. 10: pp. 133–134. 1966.

Chapter 24 — Chemical Stresses — Poisons, Toxins

1. M. Vauthey. Protective Effect of Vitamin C against Poisons. *Praxis* (Bern), vol. 40: pp. 284–286. 1951.

J. V. Mavin. Experimental Treatment of Acute Mercury Poisoning of Guinea Pigs with Ascorbic Acid. *Revista de la Sociedad Argentina de Biologia* (Buenos Aires), vol. 17: pp. 581–586. 1941.

M. Mokranjac and C. Petrovic. Vitamin C as an Antidote in Poisoning by Fatal Doses of Mercury. *Comptes Rendus Hebdomadaires des Séances de l'Academie des Sciences,* vol. 258: pp. 1341–1342. 1964.

D. W. Chapman and C. F. Shaffer. Mercurial Diuretics. *Archives of Internal Medicine,* vol. 79: pp. 449–456. 1947.

A. Ruskin and B. Ruskin. Effect of Mercurial Diuretics upon Respiration of Rat Heart and Kidney. III. *Texas Reports on Biology and Medicine,* vol. 10: p. 429. 1952.

2. H. N. Holmes et al. Effect of Vitamin C on Lead Poisoning. *Journal of Laboratory and Clinical Medicine,* vol. 24: pp. 1119–1127. 1939.

S. W. Marchmont-Robinson. Effect of Vitamin C on Workers Exposed to Lead Dust. *Journal of Laboratory and Clinical Medicine,* vol. 26: pp. 1478–1481. 1941.

L. Pillemer et al. Vitamin C in Chronic Lead Poisoning. *American Journal of Medical Science,* vol. 200: pp. 322–327. 1940.

H. Han-Wen et al. Treatment of Lead Poisoning. II. Experiments on the Effect of Vitamin C and Rutin. *Chinese Journal Internal Medicine,* vol. 7: pp. 19–20. 1959.

A. M. Dannenberg et al. Ascorbic Acid in the Treatment of Chronic Lead Poisoning. *Journal American Medical Association,* vol. 114: pp. 1439–1440. 1940.

G. A. Uzbekov. Ascorbic Acid and Cysteine as Detoxicants in Lead Poisoning. *Voprosy Meditsinskoi Khimii* (Moskva), vol. 6: pp. 183–187. 1960.

J. Gontzea et al. The Vitamin C Requirements of Lead Workers. *Internationale Zeitschrift fur Augenwardte Phisiologie Einschliesslich Arbeits Physiologie* (Berlin), vol. 20: pp. 20–33. 1963.

3. E. W. McChesney et al. Detoxication of Neoarsphenamine by Means of Various Organic Acids. *Journal of Pharmacology and Experimental Therapeutics,* vol. 80: pp. 81–92. 1942.

A. F. Abt. The Human Skin as an Indicator of the Detoxifying Action of Vitamin C (Ascorbic Acid) in Reactions Due to Arsenicals Used in Antisyphilitic Therapy. *U. S. Naval Medical Bulletin,* vol. 40: pp. 291–303. 1942.

K. D. Lahiri. Advancement in the Treatment of Arsenical Intolerance. *Indian Journal of Venereal Diseases and Dermatology,* vol. 9: pp. 1–2. 1943.

E. W. McChesney. Further Studies on the Detoxication of the Arsphenamines by Ascorbic Acid. *Journal of Pharmacology and Experimental Therapeutics,* vol. 84: pp. 222–235. 1945.

N. Marocco and E. Rigotti. Kidney Protective Effect of Vitamin C in Arsenic Poisoning. *Minerva Urologica,* vol. 14: pp. 207–212. 1962.

4. M. H. Samitz et al. Studies on the Prevention of Injurious Effects of Chromates in Industry. *Industrial Medicine and Surgery.* vol. 31: pp. 427–432. 1962.

M. H. Samitz et al. Ascorbic Acid in the Prevention of Chrome Dermatitis. *Archives of Environmental Health,* vol. 17: pp. 44–45. 1968.

D. J. Pirozzi et al. The Effect of Ascorbic Acid on Chrome Ulcers in Guinea Pigs. *Archives of Environmental Health,* vol. 17: pp. 178–180. 1968.

5. A. Renzo. Salts of Gold and Vitamin C. *Brasil-Medico,* vol. 51: pp. 1135–1136. 1937.

D. Peryassu. Vitamin C and the State of Intolerance to Gold, Bismuth and Arsenobenzene. *Hospital-Rio de Janeiro,* vol. 17: pp. 127–158. 1940.

6. J. B. Lurie. Benzene Intoxication and Vitamin C. *Transactions of the Association of Industrial Medical Officers,* vol. 15: pp. 78–79. 1965.

H. Thiele. Chronic Benzene Poisoning. *Pracovni Lekarstvi,* vol. 16: pp. 1–7. 1964.

S. Forssman and K. O. Frykholm. Benzene Poisoning II. *Acta Medica Scandinavia,* vol. 128: pp. 256–280. 1947.

I. M. Filipov. Effect of Low DDT Doses upon the Ascorbic Acid Biosynthesis in Rats. *Voprosy Pitaniia* (Moskva), vol. 23: pp. 70–73. 1964.

7. P. K. Dey. Protective Action of Ascorbic Acid and Its Precursors on the Convulsive and Lethal Actions of Strychnine. *Indian Journal Experimental Biology,* vol. 5: pp. 110–112. 1967. Also *Die Naturwissenschaften,* vol. 52: p. 164. 1965.

E. Schulteiss and J. Tarai. Effect of Ascorbic Acid on Side Effects Caused by Digitalis Therapy of Heart Disease of the Aged. *Zeitschrift fur die Gesamte Innere Medizin und Ihre Grenzgebiete* (Leipsig), vol. 14: pp. 267–268. 1959.

8. I. Dainow. Ascorbic Acid in the Prevention and Treatment of Accidents due to the Sulfamides. *Dermatologica* (Basle), vol. 83: pp. 43–44. 1941.

L. Pelner. Sensitivity to Sulfonamide Compounds Probably Avoided by Combined Use with Ascorbic Acid. *New York State Journal of Medicine,* vol. 43: p. 1874. 1943.

S. L. Ruskin. Vitamin C-Sulfonamide Compounds in the Healing of Wounds. *Archives of Otolaryngology,* vol. 40: pp. 115–122. 1944.

(For references to aspirin toxicity see Reference 3, Chapter 21.)

E. B. Vedder and C. Rosenberg. *Journal of Nutrition*, vol. 16: p. 57. 1938.

9. K. Hwi et al. A Study of the Therapeutic Effect of Large Dosage of Injected Ascorbic Acid on the Depression of the Central Nervous System as in Acute Poisoning due to Barbiturates. *Acta Pharmaceutica Sinica* (Peking), vol. 12: pp. 764–765. 1965.

R. Ghione. Morphine Spasm and C-Hypervitaminosis. *Vitaminologia* (Turin), vol. 16: pp. 131–136. 1958.

10. K. H. Beyer et al. The Relation of Vitamin C to Anesthesia. *Surgery, Gynecology and Obstetrics*, vol. 79: pp. 49–56. 1944.

11. P. K. Dey. Efficacy of Vitamin C in Counteracting Tetanus Toxin Toxicity. *Naturwissenschaften*, vol. 53: p. 310. 1966.

F. R. Klenner. Recent Discoveries in the Treatment of Lockjaw with Vitamin C and Tolsenol. *Tri-State Medical Journal*. July 1954.

I. Nitzesco et al. Antitoxic Powers of Vitamin C. *Bulletin Academie de Médicin de Roumanie*, vol. 3: pp. 781–782. 1938.

12. A. Buller-Souto and C. Lima. Action of Vitamin C on the Toxins of Gas Gangrene and Others. *Memorias do Institute Butantan*, vol. 12: pp. 265–296. 1938. (Also published in *Comptes Rendus des Séances de la Société de Biologie et de Ses Filiales* (Paris); See *Chemical Abstracts*, 1939.)

13. J. H. Perdomo. Snake Venom and Vitamin C. *Revista de la Faculatad de Medicina* (Bogota), vol. 15: pp. 769–772. 1947.

F. K. Khan. Antidotes of Cobra Venom. *Journal Indian Medical Association*, vol. 12: p. 313. 1943.

F. R. Klenner. The Use of Vitamin C as an Antibiotic. *Journal Applied Nutrition*, vol. 6: pp. 274–278. 1953.

W. J. McCormick. Ascorbic Acid as a Chemotherapeutic Agent. *Archives of Pediatrics*, vol. 69: pp. 151–155. 1952.

F. R. Klenner. The Black Widow Spider. *Tri-State Medical Journal*, December 1957.

14. G. Holland and W. Chlosta. Vitamin C and Mushroom Poisoning. *Deutsche Medizinische Wochenschrift*, vol. 65: p. 1852. 1939.

15. K. H. Beyer. Protective Action of Vitamin C against Experimental Hepatic Damage. *Archives Internal Medicine*, vol. 71: pp. 315–324. 1943.
    M. A. Soliman et al. Vitamin C as Prophylactic Drug Against Experimental Hepatotoxicity. *Journal Egyptian Medical Association*, vol. 48: pp. 806–812. 1965.

Chapter 25 — Physical Stresses

1. C. L. Pirani. Review: Relation of Vitamin C to Adrenocortical Function and Stress Phenomena. *Metabolism*, vol. 1: pp. 197–222. 1952.

2. J. Zook and G. R. Sharpless. Vitamin C in Artificial Fever. *Proceedings Society Experimental Biology and Medicine*, vol. 39: pp. 233–236. 1938.
    E. M. Thompson et al. The Effect of High Environmental Temperature on Basal Metabolism and Serum Ascorbic Acid Concentration of Women. *Journal of Nutrition*, vol. 68: pp. 35–47. 1959.
    A. Henschel et al. Vitamin C and Ability to Work in Hot Environments. *American Journal of Tropical Medicine*, vol. 24: pp. 259–265. 1944.
    W. L. Weaver. The Prevention of Heat Prostration by Use of Vitamin C. *Southern Medical Journal*, vol. 41: pp. 479–481. 1948.
    L. A. Shoudy and G. H. Collings, Jr. Clinical Trial of Vitamin B_1 and Vitamin C in the Prevention of Heat Disease. *Industrial Medicine*, vol. 14: pp. 573–575. 1945.
    F. T. Agarkov. New Possibilities of Increasing Heat Resistance of the Body in Light of Experimental Data. *Patologicheskaia Fiziologiia i Ekspermental'naia Terapiia* (Moskva), vol. 6: pp. 70–73. 1962.

3. D. H. Klasson. Ascorbic Acid in the Treatment of Burns. *New York State Journal of Medicine*, pp. 2388–2392. October 15, 1951.

4. F. R. Klenner. Observations on the Dose and Administration of Ascorbic Acid When Employed Beyond the Range of a Vitamin in Human Pathology. *Journal of Clinical Nutrition,* vol. 23: pp. 61–88. 1971.

5. M. B. Coventry and G. B. Logan. Emergency Treatment of Burns in Children. *Postgraduate Medicine,* vol. 15: pp. 150–156. 1954.
C. E. Emery, Jr., et al. Effect of Thermal Injury on Ascorbic Acid and Tyrosine Metabolism. *Proceedings Society Experimental Biology and Medicine,* vol. 106: pp. 267–270. 1961.
J. Kalina and B. Hejda. Vitamin C in Patients with Burns. *Acta Chirurgicae Plasticae,* vol. 7: pp. 139–145. 1965.

6. L. P. Dugal. Vitamin C in Relation to Cold Temperature Tolerance. *Annals New York Academy of Sciences,* vol. 92, Article 1: pp. 307–317. 1961.
L. P. Dugal and M. Therien. Ascorbic Acid and Acclimatization to Cold Environment. *Canadian Journal of Research,* vol. 25, Sec. E: pp. 111–136. 1947.
L. P. Dugal and G. Fortier. Ascorbic Acid and Acclimatization to Cold in Monkeys. *Journal of Applied Physiology,* vol. 5: pp. 143–146. 1952.
J. Leblanc et al. Studies on Acclimatization and on the Effect of Ascorbic Acid in Men Exposed to Cold. *Canadian Journal Biochemistry and Physiology,* vol. 32: pp. 407–427. 1954.
N. Glickman et al. The Tolerance of Man to Cold as Affected by Dietary Modifications: High Versus Low Intake of Certain Water-Soluble Vitamins. *American Journal of Physiology,* vol. 146: pp. 538–558. 1946.

7. G. Ungar. Effect of Ascorbic Acid on the Survival of Traumatized Animals. *Nature* (London), vol. 1: pp. 637–638. 1942.
W. A. Andreae and J. S. L. Browne. Ascorbic Acid Metabolism After Trauma in Man. *Canadian Medical Association Journal,* vol. 55: pp. 425–432. 1946.
M. F. Merezhinskii. Preservation of Ascorbic Acid and Glutathione Resources in Tissues of Animals Suffering from

Trauma and Supplied with Various Amounts of Vitamin C. *Chemical Abstracts*, vol. 57: pp. 15712–15713. 1962.

8. W. Pfannstiel. *Luftfahrtmed Abhandl*, vol. 2: p. 234. 1938; and G. Dorholt. Ibid. vol. 2: p. 240, 1938. Cited in Krasno et al.

J. M. Peterson. Ascorbic Acid and Resistance to Low Oxygen Tension. *Nature*, vol. 148: p. 84. 1941.

L. R. Krasno et al. Effect of Repeated Exposure of Human Subjects to 18,000 Feet Without Supplemental Oxygen. *Aviation Medicine*, vol. 21: pp. 283–292, 312. 1950.

I. Wesley et al. The Use of Vitamin C in Aviation Medicine. *Vojnosanitetski Pregled* (Beograd), vol. 16: pp. 207–211. 1959.

M. M. Brooks. Methylene Blue, an Antidote to Altitude Sickness. *Aviation Medicine*, vol. 19: pp. 298–299. 1948.

9. R. Seltser and P. E. Sartwell. The Effect of Occupational Exposure to Radiation on the Mortality of Physicians. *Journal American Medical Association*, vol. 190: pp. 90–92. 1964.

E. B. Lewis. Leukemia, Multiple Myeloma and Aplastic Anemia in American Radiologists. *Science*, vol. 142: pp. 1492–1494. 1963.

10. C. H. Kretzschmer et al. The Effect of X rays on Ascorbic Acid Concentration in Plasma and in Tissues. *British Journal of Radiology*, vol. 20: pp. 94–99. 1947.

M. M. Monier and R. J. Weiss. Increased Excretion of Dehydroascorbic Acid and Diketogulonic Acids by Rats after X-ray Irradiation. *Proceedings Society Experimental Biology and Medicine*, vol. 81: pp. 598–599. 1952.

H. L. Oster et al. Effect of Whole Body X-Irradiation on Ascorbic Acid of Rat Tissues. *Proceedings Society Experimental Biology and Medicine*, vol. 84: pp. 470–473. 1953.

A. Hochman and I. Block-Frankenthal. The Effect of Low and High X-ray Dosage on the Ascorbic Acid Content of the Suprarenal. *British Journal of Radiology*, vol. 26: pp. 599–600. 1953.

Z. Ya. Dolgova. Ascorbic Acid Exchange During the Action of X rays on the Organism. *Meditsinskaya Radiologiya* (Moskva), vol. 7: pp. 67–70. 1962.

11. C. Carrie and O. Schnettler. Prevention of Leucopenia aftei Roentgen Irradiation. *Strahlentherapie,* vol. 66: pp. 149–154. 1939.

A. Clausen. Treatment of X-ray Leucopenia with Vitamin C. *Acta Radiologica,* vol. 23: pp. 95–98. 1942.

W. S. Wallace. Studies in Radiation Sickness II. *Southern Medical Journal,* vol. 34: pp. 170–173. 1941.

V. Kalnins. The Effect of X-ray Irradiation on the Mandibles of Guinea Pigs Treated with Large and Small Doses of Ascorbic Acid. *Journal of Dental Research,* vol. 32: pp. 177–188. 1953.

V. S. Yusipov. Effect of Ascorbic Acid on the Carbohydrate Function of the Liver and the Survival Rate of Animals with Acute Radiation Sickness. *Meditsinskaia Radiologiia* (Moskva), vol. 4: p. 78. 1959.

V. S. Yusipov. The Role of Ascorbic Acid in Radiation Sickness. *Meditsinskaia Radiologiia* (Moskva), vol. 4: pp. 79–81. 1959.

12. E. Genazzani and E. Miele. Ionizing Radiations and Lysozyme. *II. Bollettino della Societa Italiana di Biologia Sperimentale* (Napoli), vol. 35: pp. 1798–1801. 1959.

B. Shapiro et al. Ascorbic Acid Protection Against Inactivation of Lysozyme and Aldolase by Ionizing Radiation. *U. S. Air Force School of Aerospace Medicine,* SAM-TR-65–71: pp. 1–3. November 1965.

B. Shapiro and G. Kollman. Protection by Ascorbic Acid Against Radiation Damage in Vitro. *Journal of the Albert Einstein Medical Center* (Philadelphia), vol. 15: pp. 63–70. 1967.

Chapter 26 — Pollution and Smoker's Scurvy

1. National Academy of Sciences. Effects of Chronic Exposure to Low Levels of Carbon Monoxide on Human Health, Behavior and Performance, Washington, D. C., p. 15. 1969.

2. J. W. Swinnerton et al. The Ocean: A Natural Source of Carbon Monoxide. *Science,* vol. 167: pp. 984–986. 1970.

3. V. M. Nizhegorodov. Effects of Chronic Carbon Mon-

oxide Poisoning on 24-Hour Vitamin C Requirements in Animals. *Zdravo-okhr* (Byeloruss), vol. 8: pp. 50-53. 1962.

F. R. Klenner. The Role of Ascorbic Acid in Therapeutics. *Tri-State Medical Journal,* November 1955.

P. P. Gray, I. Stone and H. Rothchild. The Action of Sunlight on Beer. *Wallerstein Laboratories Communications,* vol. 4: pp. 29–40. 1941.

4. G. Ungar and M. Bolgert. Attempts to Prevent Fatal Pulmonary Lesions from the Inhalation of Irritating Vapors with Ascorbic Acid and with Histaminase. *Comptes Rendus des Séances de la Société de Biologie et de Ses Filiales* (Paris), vol. 129: pp. 1107–1109. 1938.

   S. Mittler. Protection against Death due to Ozone Poisoning. *Nature,* vol. 181: pp. 1063–1964. 1958.

5. L. H. Strauss and P. Scheer. Effect of Nicotine on Vitamin C Metabolism. *International Zeitschrift fur Vitaminforschung,* vol. 9: pp. 39-48. 1939.

   W. J. McCormick. Ascorbic Acid as a Chemotherapeutic Agent. *Archives Pediatrics,* vol. 69: pp. 151–155. 1952.

   A. Bourquin and E. Musmanno. Effect of Smoking on the Ascorbic Acid Content of Whole Blood. *American Journal Digestive Diseases,* vol. 20: pp. 75–77. 1953.

   S. A. Andrzejewski. Studies on the Toxicity of Tobacco and Tobacco Smoke. *Acta Medica Polona,* vol. 5: pp. 407–408. 1966.

   C. Goyanna. Tobacco and Vitamin C. *Brasil Medico,* vol. 69: pp. 173–177. 1955.

   G. Dietrich and M. Büchner. Contribution to the Vitamin C Metabolism of Smokers. *Deutsche Gesundeheitwesen,* vol. 15: pp. 2494–2495. 1960.

   C1. H. Durand et al. Latent Hypovitaminosis and Tobacco. *Concourse Medicale,* vol. 84: pp. 4801–4806. 1962.

   J. H. Calder, R. C. Curtis and H. Fore. Comparison of the Vitamin C in Plasma and Leukocytes of Smokers and Non-smokers. *Lancet,* vol. 1: p. 556. 1963.

   Z. M. Rupniewska. Duration of Smoking and Content of Ascorbic Acid in the Body. *Polski Tygodnik Lekarski* (Warszawa), vol. 20: pp. 1069–1071. 1965.

   M. Brook and J. J. Grimshaw. Vitamin C Concentration of

Plasma and Leucocytes as Related to Smoking Habit, Age, and Sex of Humans. *American Journal of Clinical Nutrition*, vol. 21 : pp. 1254–1258. 1968.

O. Pelletier. Smoking and Vitamin C Levels in Humans. *American Journal of Chemical Nutrition*, vol. 21 : pp. 1259–1267.

6. J. U. Schlegel et al. Studies on the Etiology and Prevention of Bladder Carcinoma. *Journal of Urology*, vol. 101: pp. 317–324. 1969.

Ascorbic Acid: An Anticancer Vitamin? *Medical World News*, p. 24. June 21, 1968.

Chapter 27 — Wounds, Bone Fractures, and Shock

1. Scientific Conference on Vitamin C. *Annals New York Academy of Sciences*, vol. 92, Article 1. 1961.

A. F. Abt and S. von Schuching. Catabolism of L-Ascorbic-I-C[14] Acid as a Measure of its Utilization in the Intact and Wounded Guinea Pig on Scorbutic Maintenance and Saturation Diets. *Annals New York Academy of Sciences*, vol. 92: pp. 148–158. 1961.

W. van B. Robertson. The Biochemical Role of Ascorbic Acid in Connective Tissue. *Annals New York Academy of Sciences*, vol. 92: pp. 159–167. 1961.

B. S. Gould. Ascorbic Acid-Independent and Ascorbic Acid-Dependent Collagen-Forming Mechanisms. *Annals New York Academy of Sciences*, vol. 92: pp. 168–174. 1961.

J. H. Crandon et al. Ascorbic Acid Economy in Surgical Patients. *Annals New York Academy of Sciences*, vol. 92: pp. 246–267. 1961.

H. M Fullmer et al. Role of Ascorbic Acid in the Formation and Maintenance of Dental Structures. *Annals New York Academy of Sciences*, vol. 92: pp. 286–294. 1961.

R. E. Lee. Ascorbic Acid and the Peripheral Vascular System. *Annals New York Academy of Sciences*, vol. 92: pp. 295–301. 1961.

Personal communication from Dr. Marvin D. Steinberg, Director, Department of Podiatry, Jewish Memorial Hospital, New York, New York.

2. B. Chakrabarti and S. Banerjee. Dehydroascorbic Acid Level in Blood of Patients Suffering from Various Infectious Diseases. *Proceedings Society Experimental Biology and Medicine,* vol. 88: pp. 581–583. 1955.

   A. Hoffer and H. Osmond. Scurvy and Schizophrenia. *Diseases of the Nervous System,* vol. 24: pp. 1-12. May 1963.

3. J. N. Bhaduri and S. Banerjee. Ascorbic Acid, Dehydroascorbic Acid and Glutathione Levels in Blood of Patients Suffering from Infectious Diseases. *Indian Journal of Medical Research,* vol. 48: pp. 208–211. 1960.

4. G. Ungar. Effect of Ascorbic Acid on the Survival of Traumatized Animals. *Nature,* vol. 149: pp. 637–638. 1942.

   G. Ungar. Experimental Traumatic "Shock." *Lancet,* vol. 1: pp. 421–424. 1943.

   C. P. Stewart et al. Intravenous Ascorbic Acid in Experimental Acute Haemorrhage. *Lancet,* vol. 1: pp. 818–820. 1941.

   E. McDevitt et al. Vitamin C in Peripheral Vascular Failure. *Southern Medical Journal,* vol. 37: pp. 208–211. 1944.

   C. D. de Pasqualini. The Effect of Ascorbic Acid on Hemorrhagic Shock in the Guinea Pig. *American Journal of Physiology,* vol. 147: pp. 598–601. 1946.

5. H. N. Holmes. The Use of Vitamin C in Traumatic Shock. *The Ohio State Medical Journal,* vol. 42: pp. 1261–1264. 1946.

6. S. M. Levenson et al. Ascorbic Acid, Riboflavin, Thiamin and Nicotinic Acid in Relation to Severe Injury, Hemorrhage and Infection in the Human. *Annals of Surgery,* vol. 124: pp. 840–856. 1946.

   F. A. Simeone. Hemorrhagic Shock: Metabolic Effects. *Science,* vol. 141: pp. 536–542. 1963.

7. E. deJ. Zerbini. Vitamin C in Gastric Resection for Peptic Ulcer. *Archives of Surgery,* vol. 54: pp. 117–120. 1947.

   Z. Pataky, et al. Vitamin C in the Control and Prevention of Surgical Shock. *Zentralblatt fur Chirurgie,* vol. 82: pp. 883–887. 1957.

   L. A. Kashchevskaia. Dynamics of Blood Ascorbic Acid in

State of Shock. *Biulleten Eksperimental 'noi Biologii i Meditsiny* (Moskva), vol. 42: pp. 60–66. 1957.

8. J. G. Strawitz et al. The Effect of Methylene Blue and Ascorbic Acid in Hemorrhagic Shock. *Surgical Forum,* vol. 9: pp. 54–58. 1958.

9. J. A. Santomé and O. A. Gomez. Ascorbic Acid and Hemorrhagic Shock. I. Changes in Plasma and Whole Blood. *Acta Physiologica Latino-Americana,* vol. 13: pp. 150–154. 1963. II. Changes in the Whole Adrenal Gland and in the Adrenal Cortex. *Acta Physiologica Latino-Americana,* vol. 13: pp. 155–158. 1963.
G. Kocsard-Varo. The Physiologic Role of Adrenalin, Nor-Adrenalin and Vitamin C in Homeostasis. *Journal Oto-Laryngological Society of Australia* (Melbourne), vol. 2: pp. 68–74. 1967.

10. I. Gore et al. Capillary Hemorrhage in Ascorbic Acid-Deficient Guinea Pigs. Ultrastructural Basis. *Archives of Pathology,* vol. 85: pp. 493–502. 1968.

11. M. H. Weil and H. Shubin. The "VIP" Approach to the Bedside Management of Shock. *Journal American Medical Association,* vol. 207: pp. 337–340. 1969.

Chapter 28 — Pregnancy

1. E. L. Kennaway and M. M. Tipler. The Ascorbic Acid Content of the Liver in Pregnant Rats. *British Journal of Experimental Biology,* vol. 28: pp. 351–353. 1947.
Food and Nutrition Board, National Academy of Sciences. *Recommended Dietary Allowances,* Seventh Revised Edition, Washington, D.C. 1968.
T. H. Ingalls. Ascorbic Acid Requirements in Early Infancy. *New England Journal of Medicine,* vol. 218: pp. 872–875. 1938.
C. E. Snelling and S. H. Jackson. Blood Studies of Vitamin C During Pregnancy, Birth and Early Infancy. *Journal of Pediatrics,* vol. 14: pp. 447–451. 1939.

2. A. Ingier. A Study of Barlow's Disease Experimentally

Produced in Fetal and Newborn Guinea Pigs. *Journal of Experimental Medicine*, vol. 24: pp. 525–539. 1915.

O. B. Saffry and J. C. Finerty. Injection of Corpora Lutea Extract in Pregnant Guinea Pigs on a Vitamin C-Limited Diet. *Transactions Kansas Academy of Science*, vol. 42: pp. 483–485. 1939.

M. M. Kramer et al. Disturbances of Reproduction and Ovarian Changes in the Guinea Pig in Relation to Vitamin C Deficiency. *American Journal Of Physiology*, vol. 106: pp. 611–622. 1933.

M. Goettsch. Relationship Between Vitamin C and Some Phases of Reproduction in the Guinea Pig. *American Journal of Physiology*, vol. 95: pp. 64–70. 1930.

3. K. D. Paeschke and H. W. Vasterling. Photometrischer Askorbinsaure-Test zur Bestimmung der Ovulation. *Zentralblatt fur Gynakologie*, vol. 24: pp. 817–820. 1968.

A. P. Pillay. Vitamin C and Ovulation. *Indian Medical Gazette*, vol. 75: pp. 91–93. 1940.

C. Bertetti and C. Nonnis-Marzano. On the Biological Importance of Ascorbic Acid During Vitellogenesis of the Human Egg. *Biologica Latina* (Milano), vol. 16: pp. 77–98. 1963.

4. N. Räihä. On the Placental Transfer of Vitamin C. *Acta Physiologica Scandinavica*, vol. 45: Supplement 155: pp. 5–53. 1958.

M. P. Martin et al. The Vanderbilt Cooperative Study of Maternal and Infant Nutrition. *Journal of Nutrition*, vol. 62: pp. 201–224. 1957.

P. Pankamaa and N. Räihä. Vitamin C Deficiency as a Factor Influencing Seasonal Fluctuations in the Frequency of Stillbirth. *Études Néo-Natales*, vol. 6: pp. 145–148. 1957.

W. J. J. De Sauvage Nolting. Hersengroeistoornissen door Vitamin C gebrek. *Geneeskundige Gids*, vol. 3: pp. 349–351. 1955.

5. E. McDevitt et al. Selective Filtration of Vitamin C by the Placenta. *Proceedings Society for Experimental Biology and Medicine*, vol. 51: pp. 289–290. 1942.

C. P. Manahan and N. J. Eastman. The Cevitamic Acid

Content of Fetal Blood. *Bulletin Johns Hopkins Hospital*, vol. 62: pp. 478–481. 1938.

R. L. Mindlin. Variations in the Concentration of Ascorbic Acid in the Plasma of the Newborn Infant. *Journal of Pediatrics*, vol. 16: pp. 275–284. 1940.

L. B. Slobody et al. A Comparison of the Vitamin C in Mothers and Their Newborn Infants. *Journal of Pediatrics*, vol. 29: pp. 41–44. 1946.

H. M. Teel et al. Vitamin C in Human Pregnancy and Lactation. *American Journal Diseases of Children*, vol. 56: pp. 1004–1010. 1938.

D. Jackson and E. A. Park. Congenital Scurvy. *Journal of Pediatrics*, vol. 7: pp. 741–753. 1935.

6. L. Ley. Therapy of Habitual Abortion with Vitamin C. *Münchener Medizinische Wochenschrift*, vol. 84: pp. 1814–1816. 1937.

H. Teil. Can Hypovitaminosis C Cause Habitual Abortion? *Zentrallblatt fur Gynakologie*, vol. 63: pp. 1784–1792, 1838–1844. 1939.

C. T. Javert and H. J. Stander. Plasma Vitamin C and Prothrombin Concentration in Pregnancy and in Treatment, Spontaneous and Habitual Abortion. *Surgery, Gynecology and Obstetrics*, vol. 75: pp. 115–122. 1943.

W. E. King. Vitamin Studies in Abortions. *Surgery, Gynecology and Obstetrics*, vol. 80: pp. 139–142. 1945.

R. B. Greenblatt. Habitual Abortion. *Obstetrics and Gynecology*, vol. 2: pp. 530–534. 1953.

L. V. Dill. Therapy of Late Abortion. *Medical Annals* (District of Columbia), vol. 23: pp. 667–669. 1954.

C. T. Javert. Pathology of Spontaneous Abortion II. Relationship of Decidual Hemorrhage to Spontaneous Abortion and Vitamin C Deficiency. *Texas State Journal of Medicine*, vol. 50: pp. 652–657. 1954.

C. T. Javert. Repeated Abortion. *Obstetrics and Gynecology*, vol. 3: pp. 420–434. 1954.

G. W. Preuter. A Treatment for Excessive Uterine Bleeding. *Applied Therapeutics*, vol. 3: pp. 351–355. 1961.

G. L. Wideman et al. Ascorbic Acid Deficiency and Premature Rupture of Fetal Membranes. *American Journal of Obstetrics and Gynecology*, vol. 88: pp. 592–595. 1964.

7. P. H. Phillips et al. The Relationship of Ascorbic Acid to Reproduction in the Cow. *Journal of Dairy Sciences,* vol. 24: pp. 153–158. 1941.

8. W. Neuweiler. Hypervitaminosis and Its Relation to Pregnancy. *International Zeitschrift fur Vitaminforschung,* vol. 22: pp. 392–396. 1951.
   G. Mouriquand and V. Edel. On Hypervitaminosis C. *Comptes Rendus de la Société de Biologie de Lyon,* vol. 147: pp. 1432–1434. 1953.

9. M. P. Lamden and C. E. Schweiker. Effects of Prolonged Massive Administration of Ascorbic Acid to Guinea Pigs. *Federation Proceedings,* vol. 14: pp. 439–440. 1955.
   M. L. Steel Growth and Reproduction of Guinea Pigs Fed Three Levels of Ascorbic Acid. Ph.D. thesis, Cornell University, September 1968.
   C. G. King. Ascorbic Acid Intake and Viable Young of Guinea Pigs. *Proceedings 7th International Congress of Nutrition,* vol. 5: p. 595. 1967.

10. E. P. Samborskaia. Characteristics of the Effect of Ascorbic Acid on the Reproductive System of Laboratory Animals. *Biulleten Eksperimental 'noi Biologii i Meditsiny* (Moskva), vol. 54: pp. 110–114. 1962.
    E. P. Samborskaia. Effect of Large Doses of Ascorbic Acid on Course of Pregnancy in the Guinea Pig. *Biulleten Eksperimental 'noi Biologii i Meditsiny,* vol. 57: pp. 105–108. 1964.
    E. P. Samborskaia. The Mechanism of Artificial Abortion by the Use of Ascorbic Acid. *Biulleten Eksperimental 'noi Biologii i Meditsiny,* vol. 62: pp. 96–98. 1966.
    H. A. Pearse and J. D. Trisler. A Rational Approach to the Treatment of Habitual Abortion and Menometrorrhagia. *Clinical Medicine,* vol. 4: pp. 1081-1084. 1957.
    H. Ainslee. Treatment of Threatened Abortion. *Obstetrics and Gynecology,* vol. 13: pp. 185–189. 1959.

11. F. R. Klenner. Observations on the Dose and Administration of Ascorbic Acid When Employed Beyond the Range of a Vitamin in Human Pathology. *Journal of Applied Nutrition,* vol. 23: pp. 61–88. 1971.

12. W. Spitzer. Oxytocic Action of Ascorbic Acid. *British Medical Journal*, vol. 2: pp. 976–977. 1947.

    H. Tasch. Relation between Ascorbic Acid and Laboi Pains. *Zentralblatt fur Gynakologie*, vol. 73: pp. 999–1008. 1951.

    W. J. McCormick. The Striae of Pregnancy: A New Etiological Concept. *L'Union Médicale du Canada*, vol. 77: pp. 916–920. 1948.

13. M. LeCoq. Vitamin C and Dysmenorrhea. *Gazette Médicale de France*, vol. 67: pp. 1111–1112. 1960.

14. E. Derankova. Therapy of Gynecologic Hemorrhages. *Sovetskoe Vrachebnoe Zhurnal*, vol. 42: pp. 25–28. 1938.

    G. E. Morris. Hyperhemorrhea due to Scurvy. *Post Graduate Medicine*, vol. 14: pp. 443–445. 1953.

    J. D. Cohen and H. W. Rubin. Functional Menorrhagia. *Current Therapeutic Research*, vol. 2: pp. 539–542. 1960.

    Annotations. Menorrhagia. *Lancet*, vol. 1: pp. 1090–1091. 1963.

15. L. Bonnin. Augmentation of Stilbesterol Effect in Menopausal Women by Vitamin C. *New York State Journal of Medicine*, vol. 45: pp. 895–896. 1945.

    C. J. Smith. Non-Hormonal Control of Vaso-Motor Flushing in Menopausal Patients. *Chicago Medicine*, vol. 67: pp. 193–195. 1964.

Chapter 29 — Mental Disease

1. Newsletter, American Schizophrenia Foundation, Octobei 1967.

2. J. L. W. Thudichum. *A Treatise on the Chemical Constitution of the Brain.* London: Balliere, Tindall and Cox, 1884.

3. K. Wacholder. To What Extent is Vitamin C of Interest in Neurology and Psychiatry? *Fortschrift der Neurologie, Psychiatrie und Ihrer Grenzgebiete* (Stuttgart), vol. 10: pp. 260–288. 1938.

    F. Lucksch. Vitamin C and Schizophrenia. *Wiener Klinischer-Wochenschrift*, vol. 53: pp. 1009–1011. 1940.

    Z. A. Soloveva. Ascorbic Acid Therapy of Asthenic Depressive States. *Zhurnal Neuropathologii i Psikhiatrii imeni S. S. Korsakova* (Moskva), vol. 9: pp. 52–56. 1940.

W. A. Caldwell and S. W. Hardwick. Vitamin Deficiency and Psychoses. *Journal of Mental Science*, vol. 90: pp. 95–108. 1944.

E. Low-Maus. Vitamin C and the Nervous System. *Medicina Clinica* (Barcelona), vol. 19: pp. 299–303. 1952.

P. Berkenau. Vitamin C in Senile Psychoses. *Journal of Mental Science*, vol. 86: pp. 675. 1940.

4. W. J. J. De Sauvage Nolting. Vitamin C and Schizophrenia. *Geneeskundige Gids*, vol. 31: pp. 424–425. 1953.

W. J. J. De Sauvage Nolting. Is There a Relationship Between Psychopathy and Vitamin C? *Geneeskundige Gids*, vol. 32: pp. 269–271. 1954.

W. J. J. De Sauvage Nolting. Influence of Vitamin C on Development of Mental Disorders and Feeble-Mindedness. *Geneeskundige Gids*, vol. 33: pp. 115–118. 1955.

W. J. J. De Sauvage Nolting. Role of Vitamin C in Etiology of Mental Disease. *Geneeskundige Gids*, vol. 33: pp. 349–351. 1955.

A. G. Ramsay et al. The Vitamin C Nutritional Status and Capillary Fragility in Chronic Mental Patients. *Journal of Gerontology*, vol. 12: pp. 39–43. 1957.

B. D. Punekar. Blood Ascorbic Acid Levels of Mental Patients in Different Age Groups: Clinical Categories and Economic Status. *Indian Journal of Medical Research*, vol. 49: pp. 828–833. 1961.

N. W. De Smit and C. De Waart. Relation Between Puerperal Amentia and Plasma Level of Ascorbic Acid. *Nederlands Tijdschrift voor Geneeskunde* (Amsterdam), vol. 106: pp. 159–162. 1962.

M. H. Briggs et al. Comparison of the Metabolism of Ascorbic Acid in Schizophrenia, Pregnancy and in Normal Subjects. *New Zealand Medical Journal*, vol. 61: pp. 555–558. 1962.

A. Hoffer and H. Osmond. Scurvy and Schizophrenia. *Diseases of the Nervous System*, vol. 24: pp. 273–285. 1963.

G. Milner. Ascorbic Acid in Chronic Psychiatric Patients— A Controlled Trial. *British Journal of Psychiatry*, vol. 109: pp. 294–299. 1963.

S. Slowik. Ascorbic Acid Levels in Body Fluids of Chronic Schizophrenics. *Neurologia, Neurochirurgia i Psychiatria Polska,* vol. 15: pp. 881–887. 1965.

M. Andren-Sandberg and S. Rayner. Experiments with a Vitamin C-Containing Drink in a Mental Hospital. *Nordisk Medecin,* vol. 74: pp. 1022–1023. 1965.

A. W. Griffiths. Ascorbic Acid Nutrition in Mentally Subnormal Patients. *Journal of Mental Deficiency Research,* vol. 10: pp. 94–104. 1966.

6. H. VanderKamp. A Biochemical Abnormality in Schizophrenia Involving Ascorbic Acid. *International Journal of Neuropsychiatry,* vol. 2: pp. 204–206. 1966.

7. A bibliography of 196 references containing, among others, the papers of the Hoffer group up to 1961 appeared in the *Journal of Neuropsychiatry,* vol. 2: pp. 371–374. 1961.

8. H. Osmond and A. Hoffer. A Brief Account of the Saskatchewan Research in Psychiatry. *Journal of Neuropsychiatry,* vol. 2: pp. 287–291. 1961.

9. J. Huxley et al. Schizophrenia as a Genetic Morphism. *Nature,* vol. 204: pp. 220–221. 1964.

10. L. Pauling. Orthomolecular Somatic and Psychiatric Medicine. *Zeitschrift Vitalstoffe-Zivilisationskrankeheiten,* H. I. 1968.

    L. Pauling. Orthomolecular Psychiatry. *Science,* vol. 160: pp. 265–271. 1968.

    L. Pauling. Conference On Social Psychiatry. As reprinted in *Time,* p. 41. August 22, 1969.

11. A. A. Boulton. Biochemical Research in Schizophrenia. *Nature,* vol. 231: pp. 22–28. 1971.

Chapter 30 — The Future

1. Y. Hirata and K. Suzuki. A New Information Concerning Progressive Muscular Atrophy and Vitamin C. *Oriental Journal of Diseases of Infants,* vol. 18: pp. 83–86. 1935.

E. Y. Williams. Treatment of Multiple Sclerosis *Medical Record,* vol. 160: pp. 661–663. 1947.
L. J. Cass et al. Chronic Disease and Vitamin C. *Geriatrics,* vol. 9: pp. 375–380 (especially pp. 377 and 379). 1954.

2. J. Adam. Meniere's Syndrome and Avitaminosis. *Journal of Laryngology and Otology,* vol. 54: pp. 256–258. 1939.
H. Ohnell. Scorbutic Vertigo. *Gastroenterology,* vol. 71: pp. 129–141. 1946.
M. Atkinson. Meniere's Syndrome. *Archives of Otolaryngology,* vol. 51: pp. 149–164. 1950.

3. J. W. Norcross. Hemophilia and Avitaminosis C. *Lahey Clinic Bulletin,* vol. 2: pp. 219–222. 1942.

4. S. Mauer, et al. Effect of L-Cevitamic Acid on Insomnia. *Illinois Medical Journal,* vol. 74: pp. 84–85. 1938.

GLOSSARY

Alloxan A derivative of uric acid having a toxic, diabetes-producing action on the pancreas.

Amino Acids Substances resulting from the digestion and breakdown of complex proteins. They are the "building blocks" of the proteins.

Antioxidant A substance that hinders oxidation or the loss of electrons; also called a reducing agent.

Antiscorbutic Ascorbic acid, the substance that prevents or cures scurvy.

Ascorbic acid A carbohydrate of unusual properties produced in the liver of most mammals. Because of a defective gene, man is unable to produce this substance. Unless he takes in an outside supply of ascorbic acid, he will be dead of scurvy in three or four months. Ascorbic acid is more commonly referred to as vitamin C.

Avitaminosis A disease caused by the lack of minute amounts of a vitamin in the diet. *See* Vitamin Deficiency and Vitamin Dependent Diseases.

Bactericidal Having the ability to kill bacteria; germicidal.

Bacteriostatic The property of being able to prevent the growth of bacteria without necessarily killing them; antiseptic.

Biochemical Individuality The large variation between a given individual of a species and the so-called average.

Chemotherapy The treatment of disease by chemicals and drugs.

Cicatrix The new tissue formed in the healing wound.

Collagen The main structural protein of the body, comprising about one-third of the protein content of the body. This is the cementing substance that holds the tissues and organs intact, forms and maintains the integrity of the vein and artery walls, lends strength and flexibility to the bones, and is the main component of scar tissue and healing wounds. The body cannot produce collagen without ascorbic acid. The most distressing symptoms of scurvy are caused by defective or absent collagen.

Cross-Linking The formation of chemical bonds between adjacent smaller molecules, cementing them together to form huge, hard, inflexible molecular complexes. In the aging process, soft, flexible collagen molecules cross-link into rigid, indurated forms.

Deficiency Disease A disease caused by the lack of an essential substance, which may be corrected by the oral intake of the essential substance.

Dehydroascorbic Acid An undesirable oxidation product of ascorbic acid. For full good health, there must be low ratios of dehydroascorbic acid, and its production in the body minimized. This is accomplished by full correction of the genetic disease hypoascorbemia.

Enzymes Highly specific catalysts, produced by plants and animals, which speed up chemical reactions. The living body contains thousands of enzymes, all doing their separate jobs simultaneously.

Free Radical A highly active intermediate found in chemical reactions, such as in the oxidation of ascorbic acid.

Glucose A normal sugar component of plants and animals, used as a source of energy.

Hemodialysis The process utilized in the artificial kidney to purify the blood of a patient with defective kidneys.

Hormones Chemical messengers produced in the body, usually in the endocrine glands, to specifically alter the activity and response of a distant organ.

Hypoascorbemia A genetic liver-enzyme disease caused by a defective gene for the enzyme L-gulonolactone oxidase. The defective gene is carried by members of the primate suborder Anthropoidea, which includes the old world monkeys, new world monkeys, apes and man. Individuals suffering from this inherited disease require outside sources of ascorbic acid or they die of scurvy.

Intraperitoneal Within the abdomen. Many test injections on experimental laboratory animals are given by this route.

Iontophoresis The use of a mild, harmless electric current to force medication into a tissue or organ, such as the eye.

Leukocytes White blood cells. Blood may be separated into clear, yellowish blood serum and the formed cellular elements. The main cellular elements are the red blood cells and lesser amounts of various types of white blood cells.

L-Gulonolactone Oxidase One of the four enzymes required to convert glucose into ascorbic acid in the mammalian liver. Humans carry a defective gene for this enzyme, and thus cannot produce ascorbic acid in their livers.

Megascorbic Prophylaxis Use of large daily intakes of ascorbic acid to prevent disease.

Megascorbic Therapy Use of massive doses of ascorbic acid to treat various disease states and pathologic conditions.

Orthomolecular Medicine The preservation of good health and the treatment of disease by varying the concentrations in the human body of substances that are normally present in the body and are required for health. Linus Pauling suggested this new concept in 1968. Megascorbic prophylaxis and therapy are branches of orthomolecular medicine.

Oxidation A chemical reaction in which there is a transfer of electrons. The reaction comprises a two-component oxidation-reduction system in which the oxidant loses electrons and the reductant gains electrons. There are many different systems like this in the living process. The O-R system dehydroascorbic acid-ascorbic acid is one of them.

Paleopathology The study of diseases in ancient populations and fossils.

Phagocytosis The ingestion and digestion of bacteria and foreign material in the blood and tissues by white blood cells. This is one of the body's defenses against infectious diseases and injuries. The extent of phagocytosis is determined by the presence and level of ascorbic acid in the blood.

Scurvy A fatal human disease caused by a lack of ascorbic acid in the body. There are two forms of the disease: 1. acute frank clinical scurvy, due to a complete lack of ascorbic acid, in which the patients show the classical symptoms of the disease and will die in three or four months after horrible suffering; 2. chronic, subclinical scurvy, due to insufficient ascorbic acid, in which the classical symptoms are not evident but the patients are in poor health and lack resistance to disease, poisons and other stresses. The incidence of frank clinical scurvy is now rather rare in the developed countries, but the chronic subclinical form is widespread among the world's populations. Scurvy is the manifestation of uncorrected hypoascorbemia.

Scurvy Grass An effective antiscorbutic known to folk medicine of the eighteenth century and before. It is a flowering plant in the same family as the cresses, cabbage, radishes and mustards.

Topical   Pertaining to a particular spot; the local, surface application of a medicine.

Virucide   An agent that neutralizes or destroys a virus.

Vitamin Deficiency Diseases and Vitamin Dependent Diseases   Vitamin deficiency diseases are caused by the lack of traces of vitamins in the diet. Dr. Leon E. Rosenberg of Yale University's School of Medicine distinguishes these diseases from what he terms "vitamin dependent diseases." Vitamin dependent diseases are hereditary defects which can be successfully relieved by certain vitamins but require huge doses, 10 to 1000 times those needed in the "deficiency" diseases.